The Ambulance Driving Handbook

Fourth edition

I0031178

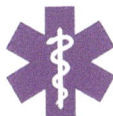

CLASS
PROFESSIONAL
PUBLISHING

Disclaimer

The Association of Ambulance Chief Executives has made every effort to ensure that the information and diagrams contained in this handbook are accurate at the time of publication. However, the handbook cannot always contain all the information necessary for determining appropriate action and cannot address all individual situations; therefore, individuals using this book must ensure they have the appropriate knowledge and skills to enable suitable interpretation.

The Association of Ambulance Chief Executives does not guarantee, and accepts no legal liability of whatever nature arising from or connected to, the accuracy, reliability, currency or completeness of the content of this handbook. Users of this handbook must always be aware that innovations or alterations after the date of publication may not be incorporated in the content. As part of its commitment to defining national standards, the Association will periodically issue updates to the content and users should ensure that they are using the most up-to-date version. Please note, however, that the Association of Ambulance Chief Executives assumes no responsibility whatsoever for the content of external resources.

It is recognised that a number of the laws in NI and Scotland differ somewhat from the laws throughout the rest of the UK; if operating in these areas then reference to these laws must be made.

Printing history

First published 2012
Second edition published 2014 (reprinted 2014)
Third edition published 2018 (reprinted 2019, 2020, 2022 and 2023)
This fourth edition published 2025

The author and publisher welcome feedback from the users of this book. Please contact the publisher:

Class Professional Publishing,
The Exchange, Express Park, Bristol Road, Bridgwater, TA6 4RR, UK.
Telephone: 01278 427800
Email: info@class.co.uk
Website: www.classprofessional.co.uk

Class Professional Publishing is an imprint of Class Publishing Ltd.
A CIP catalogue record for this book is available from the British Library.

ISBN 9781801611503 (PBK)
ISBN 9781801611510 (ePDF)
ISBN 9781801611527 (ePUB)
Designed and typeset by PHi Business Solutions
Cover design by Nicky Borowiec
Line illustrations by David Woodroffe and PHi Business Solutions
Printed in the UK by Hobbs

Refer to local recycling guidance on disposal of this book.

Product safety information can be found at https://www.classprofessional.co.uk/terms-of- use/gpsr-statement/

Contents

Foreword

Welcome to the fourth edition of *The Ambulance Driving Handbook*.

This edition has undergone a comprehensive review to include changes and definitions within the legislation, which together provide support for ambulance emergency response driver education programmes and define both vehicles and the relevant categories that the NHS statutory ambulance services utilise.

Our aim is to ensure our education programmes are delivered in a structured manner within a legal framework which supports a safe delivery system that protects the public, staff and students alike.

Emergency service drivers and attendants are required to operate under public scrutiny. As such, our aim through the use of this handbook is to guide and support safety, and provide a reference that is relevant to modern driving demands. This fourth edition is not only for the professional driver undertaking an education programme but also to act as a long term reference guide to high speed driving. The change in title reflects the broader scope of the handbook, which is now also applicable to non-emergency ambulance drivers. It supports the full spectrum of professional ambulance driving, ensuring that all drivers are equipped with a consistent and informed foundation for safe practice.

I would encourage all high-speed drivers to utilise the contents throughout your career. Ensuring we maintain a safe, structured emergency response to the public is our primary aim and through this publication we seek to enhance driver training delivery.

This book has been developed with input from sector-wide driver training specialists who have extensive knowledge and experience within the sector. As Chair of the Driver Training Advisory Group, I would like to take this opportunity to thank all the authors who have given their time and expertise so freely for the development of the publication.

Paul F. Tolley
Chair, Driver Training Advisory Group
West Midlands Ambulance Service University NHS Foundation Trust
March 2025

Acknowledgements

This handbook, along with previous editions, was initiated and developed by the Driver Training Advisory Group (DTAG) and is endorsed by the Association of Ambulance Chief Executives (AACE), which recommends its use for driver education within statutory ambulance services. The handbook was produced in consultation with UK statutory ambulance service driver training experts from the following services:

- East Midlands Ambulance Service NHS Trust
- East of England Ambulance Service NHS Trust
- London Ambulance Service NHS Trust
- NHS Isle of Wight Ambulance Service
- North East Ambulance Service NHS Foundation Trust
- North West Ambulance Service NHS Trust
- Northern Ireland Ambulance Service Health and Social Care Trust
- Scottish Ambulance Service
- South Central Ambulance Service NHS Foundation Trust
- South East Coast Ambulance Service NHS Foundation Trust
- South Western Ambulance Service NHS Foundation Trust
- Welsh Ambulance Service NHS Trust
- West Midlands Ambulance Service NHS Foundation Trust
- Yorkshire Ambulance Service NHS Trust.

Appreciation is also given to the Driver Training Advisory Group (DTAG) editorial sub-group, which undertook the review in preparation for this fourth edition, in particular Paul Tolley (WMAS), Adrian Beddow (WMAS), Ian Clark (SWASFT), Ray Edwards (WMAS), Robin Gwinnett (SWASFT), Chris Harty (SCAS), Ian Hobson (IoW), Dave Lewis (LAS), Mark McIntee (SAS), Andrew Morgan (WAST), Gavin Riddle (NEAS), Kitson Wellard (SECAmb), Angela Whyte (EEAST).

Many thanks to London Ambulance Service for the photos included in Chapter 6, West Midlands Ambulance Service NHS Foundation Trust for Figure A4.1 and South Central Ambulance Service for the cover image (reproduced with permission). Thank you also to Mark Perry from the Department of Transport for his support to ambulance service driver training, whilst bringing together this edition of the handbook.

Introduction

This handbook has been designed as a training reference to assist drivers of ambulance vehicles. It will help them to understand the standards, practices and legislation that aims to provide maximum protection to crews, passengers and other road users. It is not intended to be an exhaustive guide and should be used in conjunction with the current editions of *Roadcraft: The Police Driver's Handbook*, *The Highway Code* and *The Official DVSA Guide to Driving: The Essential Skills*.

The book makes it clear that technical mastery alone is not enough to ensure that drivers are safe; they also have to have a knowledge of legislation, of the current editions of *The Highway Code* and *Roadcraft: The Police Driver's Handbook* and of road traffic law relating to the exemptions applied to emergency response driving. This will equip drivers with the ability to interpret and modify their driving style in response to prevailing road conditions and any other hazards that may present themselves, in order to reach their destination as effectively, and as safely, as possible.

One of the main aims of this book is to minimise operational road risk and reduce undue public concern about incidents involving emergency vehicles responding to emergency calls. There are now increased possibilities for legal proceedings where there is evidence of unsafe, dangerous or careless driving, as determined by the **Road Traffic Act 1988**.

No circumstance can justify endangering lives or property by breaking the law, whether the action is exempt or not. No emergency, no matter how serious, will justify causing an accident. Emergency vehicles being driven in any situation will attract attention and, in some cases, public criticism – particularly when using emergency warning equipment. Great care and attention should be given to the manner in which you drive in order to minimise any such criticism.

This book aims to provide advice and guidance to drivers of emergency and non-emergency ambulance vehicles; for example, those undertaking non-emergency and emergency driving courses. The book can be used in a classroom environment, including a driver training unit, by those people aspiring to become an ambulance driver and prior to commencing an ambulance diving course. It should also be used by qualified drivers to maintain their professional standards and Continuing Professional Development (CPD).

CHAPTER 1

The Law

LEARNING OUTCOMES

By the end of this chapter you should:

- Understand the importance of adhering to the principles of *The Highway Code*.
- Know your responsibilities that relate to driving in a manner that does not constitute 'dangerous', 'careless' or 'inconsiderate' driving or parking.
- Know your obligations under civil law.
- Understand who is legally authorised to claim the exemption of speed according to Section 19 of the **Road Safety Act 2006**.
- Know the importance of following your trust's procedural requirements regarding motor vehicle insurance.
- Understand the Driver and Vehicle Licencing Agency's (DVLA) medical standards that must be met for different categories of driving licence, and the requirement to comply with your trust's driving licence checks.
- Know the importance and legal requirements of following your trust's road traffic collision and incident-reporting procedures.

All road users are subject to the rules of the road and the laws in relation to driving, including *The Highway Code*, the **Road Traffic Act 1988** and the **Road Safety Act 2006**. As well as being fully conversant with these, you must also understand and comply with additional legislation relating to high-speed driving, driving licences and your own medical fitness to drive.

Ambulance drivers must also comply with the policies of their individual statutory ambulance service or organisation regarding driving licence checks and their road traffic collision reporting and incident reporting procedures.

General Driving Guidelines

The Highway Code outlines the rules and guidelines that promote road safety in the UK. It is produced by HM Stationery Office in a number of formats and available to view free online. While failure to observe advice within *The Highway Code* does not render that person liable to criminal proceedings, the **Road Traffic Act 1988** (The Road Traffic (NI) Order 2007) says that any failure to adhere to the *Code*'s principles can be used to establish or negate liability in civil or criminal proceedings.

All statutory ambulance service drivers should have a sound knowledge of *The Highway Code*. It is a statutory obligation for all staff to drive in accordance with current road traffic legislation, which means that it is the responsibility of drivers to maintain their knowledge of the current edition of *The Highway Code*. You should always drive in a manner that demonstrates your skill and knowledge of driving matters to other road users in relation to the *Code*.

(!) REMEMBER

It is the responsibility of drivers to maintain their own knowledge of the current edition of *The Highway Code*.

Driving Standards Required by Law

'If a person drives a mechanically propelled vehicle on a road or other public place without due care and attention, or without reasonable consideration for other persons using the road or place, he is guilty of an offence.'

(**Road Traffic Act 1988**, amended 1991)

Civil Law

General rules, techniques and advice for all drivers and riders are contained within the current version of *The Highway Code*.

In addition to this, legislative changes that are due to be enacted will impose certain criteria on who is legally authorised to claim the exemption of speed. When enacted, Section 19 of the **Road Safety Act 2006** is likely to determine that only drivers who have satisfactorily completed a course of training in driving vehicles at high speed (exceeding the statutory speed limit) will be legally permitted to claim exemption from exceeding speed limits. In addition, they must be able to demonstrate compliance with the proposed competencies as specified in the Codes of Practice (COP).

It will be a requirement that driver competencies are assessed regularly. Similarly, instructors responsible for the delivery of this training must satisfy the COP 'instructor competencies'; these determine that the training must be carried out by appropriately qualified instructors.

Sentences for dangerous driving

In 2003, in *R v Cooksley and Others*, the Court of Appeal issued guideline penalties that should be considered when an incident results in death by dangerous driving. The Lord Chief Justice said that while jail terms should only be imposed where necessary, 'normally the only appropriate sentence to an offender found guilty of these offences is a custodial sentence'.

The Court of Appeal stated that, when determining the appropriate sentence, courts should bear in mind 'how important it is to drive home the message that dangerous driving has a potentially horrific impact'.

In a summary, the three judges said: 'Drivers must know that, if a person is killed as a result of their driving dangerously, a custodial sentence will normally be imposed no matter what the mitigating circumstances'.

This applies to all road users equally. No emergency, no matter how serious, will justify you being involved in an accident.

Motor Insurance

Statutory ambulance service employees must inform their own insurer of any road traffic collisions that they are involved in, or motoring convictions received while driving during their work activities. Failure to do so may result in your insurance being declared void by your insurers as you will have failed to disclose your full driving history.

If you receive penalty points or convictions while not at work, you must inform your employer as per local guidelines.

Collisions involving ambulances

During the 2023/24 reporting period there were 11,000 vehicle collisions reported to the insurer of UK NHS ambulance trusts, which is equivalent to 30 reported collisions per day. The most reported type of collision was ambulance vehicles hitting immobile property.

Collisions at junctions accounted for only 0.81 per cent of reported incidents but were responsible for the highest average cost per incident. This highlights the vulnerability of ambulance vehicles at junctions.

Insurance claims against UK NHS ambulance trusts in 2023/24 amounted to £22,126,073.

Clearly, cost is not the only important factor to note in vehicle collisions; there is also the associated injury to driver and third party, as well as the vehicle downtime for repair. But the statistics above clearly demonstrate the importance of diligent vehicle control and a cautious approach to the task of driving ambulance vehicles, particularly when undertaking emergency response driving.

Licence Categories C1 and D1

Most statutory ambulance services operate category C1 vehicles (which weigh between 3,500 kg and 7,500 kg) and category D1 vehicles (with 9 to 16 passenger seats).

The Driver and Vehicle Licensing Agency specifies medical standards for different groups of drivers:

- **Group 1:** drivers of motor cars and motorcycles
- **Group 2:** drivers of lorries and buses including category C1 and D1 vehicles.

These categories are either held by individuals under implied rights or are attained through licence acquisition by way of theory and practical tests depending on the year the learner driving test was passed.

Drivers who obtained entitlement to Group 1 category B (motor car) before 1 January 1997 have an automatic entitlement to category C1 and D1. Holders of C1 and D1 (minibuses for up to 16 passengers) entitlement retain this until their licence expires or is medically revoked. On renewal, the higher medical standards required for Group 2 will apply.

Legislation on driver licensing is often reviewed, and changes and amendments could be made. It is vitally important that you keep yourself up to date with any potential changes.

C1 and D1 Licence Holders Passing Tests after 19 January 2013

If you passed your driving test in any of the Group 2 licence categories after 19 January 2013, you will receive a licence, which is valid for a maximum of five years. Every five years up to the age of 45, you will sign a declaration of fitness to drive.

After you turn 45, you will need to provide a medical examination report every five years to renew your driving entitlement (www.gov.uk).

C1 and D1 Licence Holders Passing their Test before 19 January 2013

Drivers under 45 years old

If you passed a driving test in any of the Group 2 licence categories before 19 January 2013, you will come under the new rules when you renew your driving licence.

If you apply to replace your licence because it has been lost or stolen, or your personal details have changed, your new licence will run until the end of your original period. However, if you update your photo at the same time, you will come under the new five-year rule.

Drivers over 45 years old

Drivers over 45 years of age will continue to renew their entitlement as they do now. When you renew your licence at the end of a five-year period, you will need to provide a medical examination report.

More information can be found on the DVLA website (www.gov.uk).

International Restrictions

To apply for a GB driving test and obtain a full licence, you must usually be a resident of Great Britain. If you have recently moved from an EC/EEA country, you must have lived in GB for at least 185 days within the last 12 months before applying. The Immigration Act sets out the residence requirements for driving licence applications, which can be reviewed here: https://www.legislation.gov.uk/ukpga/2014/22/part/3/chapter/2/crossheading/driving-licences/enacted.

If you were a UK resident for 185 days when applying for a provisional licence, you are eligible to take both the theory and practical driving tests. The residency declaration clarifies that 'normal residence' refers to the place where you usually live, and those moving from an EC/EEA country must meet the 185-day requirement before obtaining a first full licence. Further details on driving in the UK with a non-GB licence can be found here: https://www.gov.uk/driving-nongb-licence.

Assessing medical fitness to drive

It is your responsibility to ensure you are medically fit to drive. Drivers must update the DVLA and their employer if their health needs change. Ordinarily you would need to meet blue light C1 licensing requirements and you must comply with regional guidance.

Driving Licence Checks

Ambulance services have a duty to check the driving licences of all staff who drive service vehicles. These checks take place on a regular basis, normally annually (refer to local procedures).

It is the individual licence holder's responsibility to ensure that their driving licence is valid and in date. Photo card driving licences are only valid for ten years – section 4b on the photo card provides the expiry date. The DVLA issues reminders for this.

ⓘ REMEMBER

It is your responsibility to ensure that your driving licence is valid. If you change your name or address you must inform the DVLA.

Road Traffic Collision Reporting and Incident-Reporting Procedures

Each ambulance service has individual procedures in place for reporting incidents involving motor vehicles. Drivers of service vehicles should ensure full compliance with local procedures and, above all, be fully conversant with the legal requirements of being involved in an accident as detailed in Section 170 of the **Road Traffic Act 1988**.

ⓘ KNOWLEDGE RECAP

1   Why is it important to comply with the requirements of *The Highway Code*?
2   Why is it necessary to inform your own insurer of any road traffic collision that you are involved in while driving an emergency response vehicle for your service?
3   You have to sign a declaration to show that you still meet the required medical standards when your C1 and D1 driving licence is renewed. How does this change when you reach the age of 45?
4   Whose responsibility is it to ensure that your driving licence is valid and in date?

CHAPTER 2

Driver Characteristics and Responsibilities

LEARNING OUTCOMES

By the end of this chapter you should:

- Know the specialist skills required by emergency response drivers.
- Understand how driver attitudes and behaviour can contribute to increased risk.
- Recognise how intrusive thoughts can influence the decision-making process.
- Recognise the different operational driving stress factors that may impact on emergency response drivers and how their effects can be combated.
- Recognise how passenger comfort can be compromised and the driver's responsibility to prevent this.

It is well known that human factors are a significant contributing factor to most road traffic collisions. Emergency response drivers need to demonstrate the highest standards and must be appropriately trained to deal with these factors when driving under emergency conditions.

This chapter considers some of the skills and behaviours essential for an emergency response driver as well as the stress factors that can impact on how drivers carry out their duties. It also covers drivers' responsibilities for ensuring the comfort of their passengers.

Driving Skills

There are a number of important elements in ambulance driving. You should possess the ability to:

- Manage several complicated tasks simultaneously and to a high standard
- Spread your attention during a complex drive to be able to deal with conditions in a systematic way
- Build up awareness of the whole environment
- Plan accurately and quickly
- Anticipate problems based on observations and experience
- Make sound judgements in all circumstances
- Remain alert and vigilant to ensure no hazard is overlooked.

Goals for Driver Education

In respect of standard and emergency response driving, the Goals for Driver Education (Appendix 5) represent an essential appreciation of how to structure and understand more clearly what competencies a safe driver needs and how well they will perform. Driving tasks can be described within a hierarchical framework of behaviour, conduct, competencies and decisions in a varying number of situations at different levels, within a range of driving situations.

Recognising risk is something that underpins driver education. It is important that you are aware of how physical influences of road conditions affect a vehicle and its handling and that you are cognisant of a vehicle's controls and handling characteristics.

Poor driver attitudes and behaviours may undermine the reputation of the ambulance service. The following factors may be influential to poor driving standards:

- Medical conditions
- Stressful situations

- Operational pressures
- Fatigue
- Traffic situations
- Driving at night time
- Driving in difficult weather situations.

Ambulance drivers should notify team leaders, supervisors or managers if any of these factors affect them. It is important that you are able to dynamically self-assess your actions and performance. This will help you to meet the changing circumstances and pressures you will face in your decisions and actions, especially when driving to incidents, when working extended hours or during challenging situations.

Ambulance drivers may fall short of standards because of human failings and can require a measured or bespoke intervention within the structure of ambulance driver training in order to address areas of development.

As there is no predetermined procedure for every conceivable type of situation that develops, drivers must continually perform a dynamic risk assessment on the changing environment and conditions.

You must be fully aware that attitudes related to driving under emergency response conditions may be influenced considerably by reduced concentration and intrusive thoughts, however insignificant they may seem. Examples may include, but are not limited to, focusing on the potential incident that is being responded to, personal influences relating to work or private life and instances of physical or mental fatigue, all of which can compromise the decision-making process.

A robust driving response system needs to be employed to help equip the driver with the ability to perform safely regardless of outside influences. You must bear in mind that you may be liable to prosecution if your driving falls below a safe standard. Driving commentary is an effective tool to help develop situational awareness, anticipation planning and preparation (see Chapter 16).

Training and equipment

The diverse range of vehicles in the statutory ambulance operational fleet will sometimes determine the necessity for additional training or even the requirement to hold certain driving licence categories (see Chapter 6). Regardless of the vehicle type, any driver responsible for a vehicle must ensure that they are appropriately trained and equipped to operate it in accordance with current legislation. The driver must be fully conversant with the vehicle controls – by performing a pre-driving check – and that they are satisfied that the vehicle is legally roadworthy by performing a vehicle daily inspection (see Chapter 3).

There has been some interesting research on how different types of emergency drivers are affected by different sources of stress (Sharp et al, 1997; Dorn, 2013). Three types were identified:

- Those for whom personal reward is the most important factor, such as a salary, fringe benefits, job security and working conditions
- Those who are people orientated, where helping the public, providing a service and working with people is most important
- Those for whom a professional career is most important, valuing the high prestige, independence and use of professional skills required by the job.

Operational Driving Stress

Poor stress-coping strategies would not only mean that you fail to manage the experience of driver stress but also may intensify it. Coping strategies for drivers are based on cognitive appraisals of the driving task, these include:

- **Emotion-focused coping:** self-criticism from the driver, which may impair driving performance through distraction and self-focus
- **Confrontive coping:** mastery of the driving challenge through self-assertion or conflict, which is a dangerous driver-coping strategy
- **Task-focused coping:** active attempts to change the external environment via a behavioural response, for example, reducing speed when driving conditions are dangerous, which is an effective coping strategy in the face of driver stress
- **Avoidance coping:** ignoring the stressor, often through self-distraction and diverting attention away from driving, which can impair performance
- **Reappraisal coping:** dealing with driver stress by re-appraising one's emotional and cognitive reactions, which tends to have a more positive influence on driving behaviour.

Risk taking in driving performance correlates with emotion-focused, confrontive, and avoidance coping strategies, whereas task-focused and reappraisal coping strategies usually lead to safer driving performance.

The first line of defence is to recognise the factors that cause stress; the second is to rely on training. Stress can be alleviated using the following measures (Sharp et al, 1997):

- Using all mental capacity available
- Using strategies that have been learned in advance
- Maintaining a high level of general health
- Learning to relax
- Approaching driving in a calm, confident manner
- Using the skills that have been learned
- Trying to share difficult decision making as a team

- Keeping problems separate from operational driving
- Not allowing previous incidents to impair judgement
- Putting minor errors to one side
- Learning to recognise stresses and adjust.

Professional support

There are many ways to deal with these stresses. Some people may be able to employ their own coping strategies – however, anyone experiencing difficulties should obtain professional help from the various agencies that are available.

Driver and Attendant's Responsibility to Ensure Passenger Safety and Comfort

Regardless of the type of driving being undertaken – whether standard or emergency response driving (ERD) – you have a responsibility to ensure that patients' and passengers' journeys are smooth and comfortable as well as safe.

Crew Resource Management (CRM) should be utilised and applied when driving as it is within the clinical arena. CRM is a management system that optimises the use of all available resources, including personnel, equipment, and procedures to enhance safety and efficiency. It emphasises the importance of non-technical skills alongside technical experience for safe and effective operations. It is designed to improved communication, teamwork, situational awareness, decision making and stress management.

Both the driver and attendant must share the responsibility of safety to other road users, patients and crew.

The attendant must not distract the driver during routine or emergency driving and should work to help them maximise forward vision (particularly with blind spots), hazard identification and navigation skills to increase situational awareness.

Maintaining a calm and focused environment within the cab of the vehicle will allow the driver to concentrate on the prevailing hazards ensuring a safe smooth journey whilst eliminating any potential of 'red mist' or distraction.

Inappropriate behaviour or distraction due to such things as background noise should be eliminated, this is sometimes known as a 'sterile environment'. The sterile environment should enhance the specific roles of the crew, ensuring they focus on the journey and eliminating any non-essential activities, maintaining safe focus on vehicle operation. This includes avoiding distractions and non-essential conversations during critical phases of the drive.

The attendant is required to monitor the actions of the driver to ensure they are driving to the required standard of competence as per the 'system of car control' police driving standard.

ⓘ REMEMBER

The clinician in charge of the patient's care should communicate with the driver about the nature of the drive that is required during transport to a place of definitive care. It is important to remember that the drive should be regarded as part of the treatment process and should be tailored to the particular patient's needs and condition.

As an example, a patient who has sustained a fracture, or is suffering from rheumatoid arthritis will be particularly susceptible to discomfort from uneven road surfaces or potholes. There are other traumatic injuries whereby erratic acceleration, harsh braking or hasty cornering can significantly influence the patient's prognosis. It should be emphasised that even in the cases not listed above, speed should not be so great that it interferes with the ongoing treatment of the patient care en route.

It can be a daunting experience for anyone travelling in the saloon of an ambulance; this is exacerbated by the lack of vision afforded, which does not allow for the anticipation of vehicle movements, which is usually experienced when travelling in a car. While engaged on emergency response driving it is useful to inform the attendant of approaching hazards that may affect vehicle movements so that they can ensure that they are safely restrained or suitably positioned.

It is therefore important that the drive is smooth and the system of car control is applied effectively, with emphasis given to good acceleration sense, early braking for hazards and the application of tapered braking.

Braking smoothly

Vary the brake pedal pressure when bringing the vehicle to a stop, this will give maximum braking control and ensure smoother stopping.

1 Gently take up the free play in the brake pedal.
2 Increase the brake pedal pressure progressively, as required, to bring the vehicle to stop.
3 Relax the brake pedal pressure as unwanted road speed is lost.
4 Release the brake pedal pressure just before stopping to ensure the vehicle stops smoothly.

Loading Patients into the Vehicle

When loading patients, consider the seating position that will afford them the most comfort. A seat directly above a wheel arch will generally be more susceptible to vibrations. Likewise, a seat on the offside of the vehicle is likely to be more comfortable due to most uneven surfaces, drain covers for example, being nearest to the kerb. Wherever the patient is seated, they should be securely fastened.

If seats in the vehicle are of different heights, try to ensure that the patient can reach the floor with their feet, enabling them to gain better stability when the vehicle is cornering, and point out any handrails that may be available to them.

Patients on a stretcher can feel vulnerable and insecure, especially as they are normally rear-facing. Ensure that they are securely fastened in with the securing belts and harnesses provided, and if their condition permits, that they are sitting up on the stretcher.

Safe in the Back

AACE have highlighted the importance of ensuring that both ambulance staff and patients are appropriately secured with seat belts and harnesses with their Safe in the Back campaign and video:

Key campaign messages:

- Patient treatment and patient safety are equally important.
- Drivers are primarily responsible for ensuring all seatbelts are fastened, but everyone must play their part.
- Challenging others who do not wear seatbelts is a good thing.

Confrontational Behaviour

For every action there is a reaction. If you react to a given driving situation unfavourably it could have disastrous consequences for yourself and others.

An example of when confrontational behaviour can arise is when you are engaged in an emergency response drive and progressing through a stream of heavy traffic.

Situations can arise when vehicles slow or become stationary, because they have seen or heard an approaching emergency vehicle and reacted accordingly.

A driver of a nearby vehicle that pulls out suddenly to overtake the slowing or stationary vehicles because they failed to hear or see the approaching emergency vehicle will have an initial reaction of a belligerent attitude towards the drivers of those vehicles.

This is further compounded by the driver realising why vehicles were slowing or stopping and their subsequent realisation that the emergency vehicle is now impeded from making safe progress. This loss of credibility in their driving capability can lead to the driver becoming confrontational, with reactions such as verbal abuse or hand gestures.

You can diffuse the situation by proceeding safely through without any further reactions to the situation.

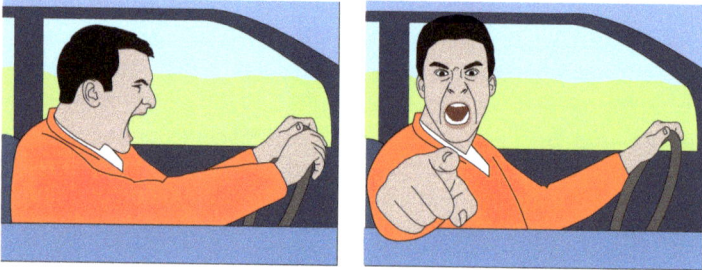

FIGURE 2.1 • Confrontational behaviour can cause severe consequences.

(?) KNOWLEDGE RECAP

1 Describe three specialist skills that emergency response drivers should possess.
2 How frequently should drivers perform dynamic risk assessments?
3 Describe two types of operational stress that drivers may encounter while carrying out their day-to-day duties.
4 Describe two methods that can be used by drivers to deal with the effects of stress.
5 Why must the comfort of patients be taken into consideration when formulating driving plans?
6 How can different seating positions within an ambulance affect passenger comfort?
7 Describe the stress coping strategies that relate to a safer driving performance.

CHAPTER 3

Vehicle Daily Inspections and Pre-Driving Checks

LEARNING OUTCOMES

By the end of this chapter you should:

- Understand why vehicle daily inspections are completed.
- Understand how often a vehicle should be inspected.
- Be able to complete a vehicle daily inspection.
- Understand why pre-driving checks are completed.
- Understand when a pre-driving check should be conducted.
- Be able to complete a pre-driving check.

This chapter outlines the various checks that are to be conducted by the driver prior to the use of any vehicle on a public road.

Why Are Vehicle Daily Inspections Completed?

Prior to the use of any vehicle for ambulance purposes, especially those utilised for response driving, comprehensive checks must be completed to ensure that those vehicles:

- Are safe for their intended use
- Are roadworthy
- Comply with all road traffic law
- Satisfy all health and safety legislation
- Set a good example to other road users.

The vehicle daily inspection (VDI) is to be conducted at the start of every shift or when there is a switch to a different vehicle during a shift.

Any defect found must be reported in compliance with the service's policy in order that such defects can be rectified. A vehicle must not be used if it does not comply with road traffic law.

Items to be Checked During Daily Inspection

1 Examination of exterior
2 Wheels and tyres
3 Under bonnet checks
4 Lights and reflectors
5 All glass, wipers and washers
6 All audible warning equipment and exhaust
7 Ambulance-specific equipment/supplies.

The checklist above is explained in more detail below in the following tables.

Examination of Exterior

TABLE 3.1 Checks for the vehicle's exterior.

What to do	Why
• As you approach the vehicle check that it sits normally on the ground. The vehicle should not be leaning to one side or sit lower to the front or rear. • Look below the vehicle for any fluids that may have been deposited on the ground. This could be water, oil or hydraulic fluid. • Check for any unrecorded damage to the bodywork. • Ensure that all body panels are in alignment and that all components (such as body panels, mirror brackets, tail lifts and locker doors) are attached securely. • Check that all doors open and close correctly. • Check that fluorescent and reflective markings or panels are clean, in good condition and undamaged.	• Adverse tilt in any direction could indicate damage to the suspension or a flat tyre. It may also indicate an incorrect loading of the vehicle. • Fluids on the ground may indicate a leak from the vehicle. Be aware that air conditioning units can expel water (this can be normal). • If you use the vehicle without identifying such damage you may be held responsible. • Any sharp edges or loose equipment can be construed as being in a 'dangerous condition'. This could lead to a prosecution under the Construction and Use Regulations. • All doors should open freely to aid exit in an emergency. • Clean panels ensure the vehicle is more conspicuous.

Wheels and Tyres

TABLE 3.2   Checks to carry out on the wheels and tyres.

What to do	Why
• Make sure that every wheel has all its wheel nuts present and that they are secure. If fitted make sure that all wheel nut security indicators are correctly aligned. • Examine for scrapes or cracks, which could weaken the wheel. • Tyre treads should be checked for their depth. Different vehicles have different legal tyre tread depths, ensure that your tyres comply. Most ambulance services will change tyres before the tread depth is less than 3 mm. • Tyres should also be checked for pressure, cuts, bulges and other damage. Check for the presence of valve caps. • Where there are twin wheels on the rear make sure there are no foreign objects wedged between their inner faces.	• Wheel damage is a possibility and a loose wheel has obvious implications. Small rust 'tracks' emanating from any of the nuts could be an indication of a loose nut. • Wheel rims are prone to damage, especially those made of metal alloys. • It is especially important to check the security of wheel nuts after a recent tyre change. • The correct depth of tread is vitally important when roads are wet, as it dispels water from the tyre road interface. • Tyre faults can lead to a catastrophic tyre failure. Some ambulance services check tyre pressures using a visual check only. Uneven tyre wear can indicate issues with the suspension.

Under Bonnet Checks

TABLE 3.3   What to look for under the bonnet.

What to do	Why
• While the vehicle is parked on a level surface, check that the engine oil, radiator coolant, power steering hydraulic fluid, brake fluid and windscreen washer levels are up towards the maximum level but not beyond. If used, exhaust additive levels (such as AdBlue) should also be checked. • Some vehicles require the engine to be warm prior to checking the dipstick – check in the vehicle's handbook. • Ambulance services have different policies that relate to who should replenish any shortfall in any of the fluid levels. • Some services have a policy where the fluids are checked by the vehicle's own diagnostic programme – this is sometimes referred to as a 'clean hands check'. • Check the security of the fuel filler cap.	• A lack of engine oil or engine coolant could result in extreme engine wear and possibly an engine seizure. This is particularly important as ambulance service vehicles have to work in arduous conditions and are sometimes in continuous use for long periods. • A low level within the brake or power steering reservoir could indicate a leak in the systems with very obvious serious consequences. • It is vitally important that only the correct oil/fluid is used to top up any levels and is best carried out by a professional mechanic.

Lights and Reflectors

TABLE 3.4   Checks for the lights and reflectors.

What to do	Why
All lights must be checked prior to using the vehicle. Those to be checked include: • Headlights: dipped, main beam, flash, flashing (if fitted) • Position lights (sidelights) front and rear • Daytime running lights • Fog lights – front and rear • Indicators front/back side repeaters/rear of mirrors • Hazard warning lights • Brake lights • Rear number plate lights • Reversing lights • Reflectors • *Emergency warning lights front/rear/side* • *Scene lighting* • *Interior lights in the cab and saloon including map-reading lights and instrument cluster lights.* Other than the items written in italics, all lights fitted must be working and clean.	• It is important to not only be able to see but also to be seen. • Vehicles with defective lighting could adversely affect the professional image of the ambulance service. • Most vehicles are able to warn the driver automatically if any of the vehicle's bulbs become defective, using a warning light on the vehicle's instrument panel. Sometimes a defective indicator bulb is highlighted by an increase in the frequency of flashes of the indicator warning light on the instrument panel.

Glass, Wipers and Washers

TABLE 3.5   Checks for all of the vehicle's glass, wipers and washers.

What to do	Why
• Ensure that the windscreen, side and rear windows are clean inside and out. Ensure that they are free of cracks or chips. • Check that the reflective surfaces of all the mirrors are clean. • Check the operation of the windscreen wipers (and rear wiper(s) – if fitted). • Check the operation of the windscreen washer (and rear washer – if fitted). Ensure the glass is wet when checking as scratching of the glass may result otherwise. • Ensure the demisters and heated windows also operate (if applicable).	• It is imperative that you are able to see clearly out of the vehicle. An extremely high proportion of driver information is derived through their eyes. • Cracks and chips can make the vehicle unfit for use and may need replacement or repair. • It is important that all-round vision is clear – this is paramount during the hours of darkness, twilight, bright sunlight and in wet conditions. • Any smears on the windscreens will limit your vision. Detergent in washer fluid will help to clean the windscreen.

Audible Warning Equipment and Exhaust

TABLE 3.6 Checking all the vehicle's audible warning equipment and exhaust.

What to do	Why
• Check that the horn, the emergency sirens and bull horn (if fitted) are operating correctly. Use the low power button, if fitted, to reduce the volume while testing. • Ensure that the vehicle's reversing alarm or warning device (if fitted) operates correctly. • Ensure that the devices warning the driver of open doors, side step deployment or rear ramp insecurity (if fitted) operate correctly. • The exhaust system should be checked to ensure that the noise emitted is not abnormally excessive and that gases are not escaping from any section of the system other than at the tail pipe. • Be aware that this should not be conducted in an enclosed space due to the toxic nature of engine exhaust gases.	• It is important that the driver checks that all audible equipment works prior to using the equipment during an emergency response.

Equipment and Supplies

TABLE 3.7 Checking all the vehicle's equipment and supplies.

What to do	Why
• Check the presence, security and function of any safety or ambulance-specific equipment. This will include such safety items as the fire extinguisher and first aid kit.	• The medical equipment and stores will be dependent on the grade of vehicle being driven.

Safety and Maintenance

Safety Notes

The person checking the lights should ensure that they do not stand directly in front or directly behind a vehicle, but safely to one side in case the driver unintentionally causes the vehicle to move. The person checking the under bonnet fluids should have possession of the ignition keys to ensure that the engine cannot be started while they are near to components that could start to move.

If the vehicle has been used just prior to the VDI being conducted, the engine compartment and exhaust system could be very hot. It is imperative that the radiator (or its header tank) filler cap is not removed if the engine is still hot, as the coolant system will be under high pressure. The release of this pressure could cause hot water and steam to be released in an explosive manner.

Many of the hydraulic fluids and oils are carcinogenic and corrosive, so skin contact must be avoided. Additionally, if any of these fluids are topped up with the incorrect fluid, damage could result.

Electric vehicles

Hybrid or electric only vehicles are becoming more popular. Their operating systems and controls are often different to regular petrol and diesel vehicle and you should ensure that you are completely familiar with their operation. Your service may provide specific information, training or guidance on how to operate them, if not then check the vehicle handbook. The handbooks of these vehicles can be used as a reference resource to establish the correct checks to be conducted.

Tyre pressures

The correct tyre pressures can be established by looking at the vehicle's handbook or are sometimes found on the rear of the fuel filling flap, attached on plates to the B pillars, or on the vehicle itself above the wheel arch.

Diesel exhaust systems

For diesel vehicles equipped with AdBlue systems, it's important to monitor the AdBlue level.

AdBlue is a non-toxic liquid that is colourless in appearance. Its purpose is to reduce harmful gases into the environment when it is introduced in microscopic form into the flow of exhaust gases. When the solution combines with exhaust emissions, it produces nitrogen and oxygen – harmless gases that occur naturally in the environment.

When a low level warning is illuminated it is important that the reservoir is replenished as soon as possible. To continue using the vehicle may eventually cause the engine management system to go into 'limp' mode. This will result in a vast reduction in engine power.

Pre-Driving Checks

The completion of a pre-driving check (PDC) will ensure that you are familiar with both the location and means of operating all the vehicle controls. It will also help to reduce driver fatigue and enhance vehicle safety.

A PDC should be completed when you first enter the vehicle. Once driven, the PDC does not need to be repeated during the shift unless another person has driven it. Throughout the shift, provided no other person has driven the vehicle, a driver only has to confirm points 1, 4 and 7.

Different vehicles may require that the list is adjusted.

Pre-Driving Checks and Order to be Checked

1   Check the parking brake is applied and check the gear lever is in neutral (manual) or the transmission is in park (automatic)
2   Adjust the position of the driver's seat and steering wheel
3   Adjust all the driver's mirrors
4   Perform the starting procedure
5   Carry out static brake tests
6   Check the auxiliary controls
7   Check the seat belts and doors
8   Carry out the moving brake test.

Parking Brake and Gear Lever

TABLE 3.8   Check parking brake is applied and familiarise yourself with gear positions.

What to do	Why
• Upon entering the vehicle, ensure that the parking brake is fully applied. • The gear lever should be checked to ensure it is in the neutral position. At this stage you should familiarise yourself with the position of each gear and be aware how to select reverse gear. You will be able to recognise that the gear lever is in the neutral position by the large amount of lateral movement available. • Automatic gearbox vehicles should have the 'Park' position selected.	• It is important to ensure that the parking brake is fully applied to ensure that it is secure. The additional weight of a person entering a vehicle could cause it to move, if on a slope. • It is imperative that the gear lever is placed in the neutral position to prevent the vehicle lurching forwards or rearwards if you were to inadvertently start the vehicle. You should be aware how to engage any chosen gear without having to look at the gear lever. • Most automatic vehicles are not able to be started if the gear selector is not in 'Park'.

Seat and Steering Wheel Positions

TABLE 3.9   Adjust position of driver's seat and steering wheel.

What to do	Why
• The driver's seat should be adjusted so that you are able to reach all the controls, be able to fully depress the driver's foot pedals and be able to use the full circumference of the steering wheel. The position must ensure a good view from the vehicle and guard against the effects of fatigue. • An ideal position can be recognised when you are able to depress the clutch fully (accelerator in automatics) and still retain a bend at the knee. When your hands are placed on the steering wheel both arms should retain a slight bend at the elbow. There are various means of adjusting a seat: • Seat height should be adjusted to ensure a clear view to the front and sides and to ensure the legs do not touch the steering wheel. • Longitudinal position of the seat base must allow you to fully depress the pedals while retaining a slight bend at the knee. • Rake angle allows the seat back to be placed to allow you to have your hands on the steering wheel at the '10 to 2' position and still retain a bend at the elbow. • Head restraint should be aligned so that the top aligns with your eye line (some vehicle's head restraints are not adjustable). • Lumbar support should be adjusted to provide support to the lower back. • The steering wheels in some vehicles allow an adjustment to their length and rake. You should combine the adjustment to compliment the seat adjustments. • Always check that the seat has located properly on its movement track to prevent movement in braking/acceleration situations.	It is important that you are able to use all the vehicle's controls. • You should not have to move position to reach any of the controls, as this could affect control of the vehicle. • It is important that the clutch pedal can be fully depressed to ensure that the drive to the transmission can be fully removed and to assist in smooth gear changes. • It is important that your hands can use the full circumference of the steering wheel, so that steering movements can be smooth and the correct degree of steering can be applied easily. • A correctly positioned seat helps to prevent driver fatigue. This, in turn, will assist you in maintaining your concentration. • In the event of a collision, the correct seating position will allow the vehicle's passive safety systems to provide you with the best possible protection and will help to mitigate injuries.

Mirror Positions

TABLE 3.10   Adjust all driver's mirrors.

What to do	Why
You should adjust the various mirrors on a vehicle to give the best possible view around the vehicle. • **Interior rear-view mirror:** take hold of the mirror frame and align it so that the entire rear window is framed. If you cannot frame the entire rear window, angle the mirror so that you can see the offside of the rear window. The top edge of the mirror should line up with the top of the rear window. In an ambulance-type vehicle, this mirror should be aligned to enable a clear view into the saloon of the ambulance. • **Exterior mirrors:** these may be adjusted by manual or electrical means. If the ignition needs to be operated, it should be switched off after the alignment has taken place. These mirrors should be aligned to show the vehicle's bodywork on the internal thirds and the other two thirds should show the view to either side of the vehicle. Ideally, you should be able to see the rear wheels or the wheel arches. The horizontal alignment should be that the rear horizon should be positioned in the centre of the mirror. • **Blind-spot or wide-angled mirrors:** these provide you with a better view of what is alongside, or sometimes in front, of the vehicle. • **Reversing cameras:** where fitted, these utilise an in-cab screen to display an image of what may be directly behind the vehicle.	• Correct alignment will allow you to achieve the best possible of the view to the side and rear of the vehicle using mirrors. However, shoulder checks are critical to eliminate the blind spots created by the vehicle's bodywork. • It is essential that you are able to see the bodywork in the mirrors, as it allows a reference as to the proximity of any object to their vehicle. • A view of the rear wheels or wheel arches also provides you with a reference to the point at which a vehicle pivots, in order to apply or remove steering accurately. • You should be aware that most mirrors distort the actual view, especially blind spot mirrors. • Reversing cameras also provide a distorted picture to the driver.

Typical features of modern mirrors

Some exterior mirrors are 'aspherical' – this is where the main part of the mirror is flat, but curves away towards the outer edge to reduce blind spots. This can cause a distorted view.

A prismatic rear-view mirror, also called a 'day/night mirror', can be tilted to reduce the brightness of lights from vehicles behind. This limits the amount of light reflected into the driver's eyes at night, but should only be used during the hours of darkness.

Modern vehicles use sensors to dim some mirrors by means of electrochromism.

Vehicle's Starting Procedure

TABLE 3.11 Carrying out all starting procedures.

What to do	Why
• The clutch pedal should be fully depressed (or an automatic gearbox placed in the 'Park' position). • Depress the footbrake repeatedly until it becomes firm and you no longer hear the vacuum within the servo being vented to atmosphere. Maintain a downward pressure on the footbrake. • Ensure all auxiliary equipment switches and other controls are in the 'off' position. • Turn the ignition key to the position that releases the steering lock, then continue to the next position until the warning lights illuminate on the instrument panel. Ensure any self-diagnostic system checks are completed (this will be model dependant). • Once all the lights have extinguished as expected, apply downward pressure to the steering wheel with the hand that is not being used to turn the key. Then rotate the ignition key until the engine starts and let the key go. • You should feel the steering wheel drop in the direction the hand is pulling and the footbrake should also drop downwards. • You should then ensure that the lights on the instrument panel extinguish, with the exception of the handbrake warning light. • If the lights do remain on, or illuminate during the journey, the vehicle should be stopped as soon as is safely possible. • Maintain downward pressure of the footbrake, but slowly raise the clutch pedal and place your left foot away from the clutch pedal. • The driver should then monitor the gauges and ensure that there is sufficient fuel for the anticipated journey.	• The clutch pedal is depressed prior to the starting procedure to prevent the vehicle moving if there is a 'false' neutral or there is a break in the linkage to the gearbox. • An additional benefit is that the starter motor only has to turn the engine, not the transmission. • The vacuum is vented within the servo to allow a check of that important system. • Ensuring all the electrical components are switched off will allow all the power of the battery to be used to start the engine. • Upon starting, the downward movement of the steering wheel indicates that the power steering pump is working correctly. The downward movement of the footbrake indicates that the servo system is working correctly. If there is not a downward movement in both of these checks, the vehicle should not be used until seen by a mechanic. • It is important to ensure that the warning lights extinguish. If they do not, you should be aware that a serious fault could have been pre-empted by the lights. To continue to drive may cause serious damage to the vehicle or render certain components inoperable. • In most ambulance services it is a disciplinary offence to run out of fuel. It could result in drastic consequences if the vehicle is en route to a serious incident or is in the process of transporting a patient to hospital.

Static Brake Tests

TABLE 3.12   Carrying out brake tests.

What to do	Why
• **Footbrake check:** with the handbrake remaining fully applied, you should allow the footbrake to rise to its original position. You should then depress the footbrake until a firm pressure is felt. The brake pedal must then be released and reapplied a total of three times. On the last application, you must maintain the downward pressure. This pressure should be firm with no further downward movement felt. • **Handbrake check:** you should ensure that the footbrake is fully applied, then fully release the handbrake to the full downward extent. This will require the pawl button to be fully depressed. You should then reapply the handbrake again, depressing the pawl button. At the top of its travel, the pawl button should then be released. You should ensure that there is no footbrake movement during the handbrake application. • **Electronic parking brake (EPR):** Refer to the vehicle's handbook to ascertain their correct operation.	• If the brake pedal maintains its pressure and no further downward 'creep' is experienced, that indicates that the hydraulic system is in good working order. • Excessive travel may indicate worn brake pads. Continued downward movement may indicate a system leak. • The handbrake check allows you to become familiar with the application and release of the handbrake. • A movement of the footbrake during the operation of the handbrake may indicate a defect with the braking system(s). • The reason that the pawl button is normally depressed when applying the handbrake is to reduce the potential wear and tear in the pawl and ratchet mechanism.

Use of pawl buttons

Some manufacturers advise that the pawl button is not depressed when applying the handbrake. Check the vehicle's handbook for advice.

Some ambulance services advise that the pawl button should not be used when conducting the static brake test and that the ratchets should be counted to indicate wear and tear on the brake cable over a period of time. However, the pawl button should always be used during normal road use to limit the amount of wear on the ratchet system.

Foot-operated parking brakes

Some vehicles are fitted with foot operated parking brakes, read the vehicle's handbook for advice on their application and release.

Parking brake use

The parking brake should not be operated when the vehicle is moving unless the primary brake system has failed. To apply the parking brake when moving could cause wheels to lock with a resulting loss of control.

Familiarity with Auxiliary Controls

TABLE 3.13   Checking the location and operation of auxiliary controls.

What to do	Why
You must systematically check all the vehicle's controls, switches and auxiliaries to ensure they are familiar with their location and method of operation. Items to locate and check the operation of include: • Climate control, air conditioning, heating and their associated vent controls • All exterior light controls – headlights, position lights, headlamp flash, indicators, hazard warning lights and fog lights • Wipers and washers (front and rear if applicable) • Heated rear window (and windscreen if applicable) • Interior lighting and map-reading lights • Audible warning instrument • Emergency equipment (lights, sirens and bull horn) • Saloon heating/lighting controls • Data terminal • Communication equipment/mobile phone hands free equipment • Satellite navigation controls • Radio and other entertainment controls • Access to storage compartments • Sun visors • Mirror adjustment controls • Central locking/release • Headlight height setting • Dimmer switch for instrument panel • Cruise controls • ESP control and any other safety systems • Lock systems and isolator switches • Emergency start button or switch.	It is critical to the safe operation of a vehicle that you are fully familiar with all the controls at their disposal. The controls should be able to be located without looking away from the road ahead. Once located, you should be proficient at operating each control. At 60 mph, for every second that elapses while you are looking for a control, the vehicle will travel roughly 30 metres. • This check of the controls is especially important when you change to a different vehicle. • While checking the controls, you should set or operate those necessary for that particular journey. • Any loose object that could prevent the application or release of the foot pedals or interferes with the vehicle's steering wheel or other controls could have catastrophic consequences. • Carpets and additional mats could also provide a source of danger if they prevent use of the foot pedals. • The manufacturer's handbook is an ideal resource to ensure familiarity with the vehicle being driven.

Seat Belts and Doors

An ambulance has numerous doors that need to be checked. Most vehicles have warning equipment to warn the driver that a door is insecure, but it is good practice to check the doors by asking all crew to check their own doors for security.

TABLE 3.14 Checking the operation of seat belts and doors.

What to do	Why

• The seat belt webbing should be fully removed from its housing to check for damage such as cuts, rips or frays.
• The webbing should be placed diagonally across the body over the shoulder to the opposite hip. There must be no twist in the webbing. The webbing should lie flat against the wearer's sternum and abdomen. The buckle should be placed into its receiving mechanism. This should then be checked to ensure that it will release the buckle and then it should be secured.
• If fitted, the seat belt height adjuster should be set so that the belt is about 25–50 mm above the shoulder.
• The seat belt inertia mechanism can be tested by pulling sharply downwards on the webbing between the housing and the user's shoulder. A sharp tug downwards should cause the mechanism to halt the deployment of any further webbing abruptly.
• Once fitted, the wearer should ensure there are no objects between the webbing and their body that may result in more serious injuries (pens, name badges etc.).
• All doors on a vehicle should be secured – it is the driver's responsibility to ensure all door security. Some ambulances have audible warnings to advise if the rear and side doors are not secure.
• Other observations that will help identify insecure doors include the illumination of the interior cab light, a kink in the smooth line of the bodywork where the door meets the main body of the vehicle when viewed through the vehicles exterior mirrors, illumination of a warning light on the vehicle dashboard, excessive road noise through partially secured doors.
• Exterior locker doors should have been checked during the PDC, however it is important that if access to these lockers has been necessary at an incident, you check their security.
	• Damage to the seat belt webbing would render the vehicle unusable until repaired.
	• It is important that seat belts are checked for wear and tear, as numerous short journeys undertaken by ambulances result in a heavy wear and tear on the seat belts. Combined with the equipment worn on the belts of clinicians, this may result in the premature wear of seat belt webbing.
	• The correct use of a seatbelt is critical in reducing or preventing injuries, should the vehicle be involved in an incident. The seat belt ensures that the occupant is in the correct position to allow the vehicle's passive safety systems to work to their maximum efficiency.
	• Passive safety systems that will benefit from the correct use of seat belts include:
	  – Airbags (front and side)
	  – Seat belt pre-tensioners
	  – Side impact protection
	  – Passenger cell protection
	  – Steering column design
	  – Whiplash protection system
	  – Head restraints
	  – Crumple zones.
	• The use of the central locking mechanism would be of benefit.

Moving Brake Test

You should be aware that adverse weather and road surface conditions will result in a longer braking distance. You must ensure there is sufficient room to carry out the moving brake test.

If there is insufficient room to conduct the test off-road, you should consider braking earlier and gently prior to the first hazard. Be aware of other road users, including cyclists and those using the footpath. Avoid conducting a moving brake test adjacent to other hazards.

TABLE 3.15 Carrying out a moving brake test.

What to do	Why
• Where possible, and prior to joining the public road, a moving brake test should be conducted. • Ideally the test should be conducted at approximately 20 mph on a level road surface in a higher gear. • Move off when it is safe to do so, announce to the vehicle occupants that you intend to conduct the test and check your mirrors to ensure it is safe to conduct the brake test. • Prior to brake application, relax your grip on the steering wheel (but be prepared to grip firmly if required), then apply the foot brake firmly and continue braking until the vehicle comes to a standstill – but not in the manner of an emergency stop. • Check that the vehicle did not deviate to the left or right and that it pulled up evenly on all four wheels within the expected distance.	• This test will confirm that the primary braking system is operating appropriately. • It is better to discover there is an issue with the brakes prior to entering a public area. • Any defect discovered will prevent the vehicle being used until repaired. • If the vehicle does not remain in a straight line, it would indicate a braking, steering, tyre or possible suspension defect. The vehicle must not be used on a public road until repaired. • If the vehicle requires a longer distance to stop than expected, it may mean that not all the brakes are operating or there is possible contamination of the brake pads/discs. • If the mobile brake test is normal you could add this to your driving commentary, stating 'the vehicle pulled up evenly on all four wheels with no adverse effects to the steering. That is hopefully the harshest braking I will have to perform today'.

Shore lines for battery charging

It is important that you ensure that the electric 'shore line' (umbilical lead) has been fully ejected before moving off. To drive off while still connected may result in extensive, and therefore expensive, damage to both the vehicle and components of the shore line equipment.

Electric plug-in vehicles might also have charging leads connected. Usually these do not self-eject when the vehicle is started. As a result, ensure that they are removed prior to activating the ignition.

Leads are often vehicle specific and may need to be taken with the vehicle – refer to your local policy.

(?) KNOWLEDGE RECAP

1 How frequently should a VDI be conducted?
2 What should you do if you find a defect during a VDI?
3 Why should vehicles be parked on a level surface when checking under-bonnet fluids?
4 How frequently should a PDC be completed?
5 State two reasons why the correct seating position is important.
6 What is a blind spot?
7 Why should the driver fully depress the clutch when starting a vehicle fitted with manual transmission?

CHAPTER 4

Reversing and Manoeuvring

LEARNING OUTCOMES

By the end of this chapter you should:

- Know the rules and advice on reversing as specified in *The Highway Code*.
- Recognise the need for teamwork.
- Understand the driver's responsibilities when carrying out low-speed manoeuvres.
- Understand the banksman's responsibilities when carrying out low-speed manoeuvres.
- Recognise and use the standard signals used to guide drivers when manoeuvring.
- Know not to solely rely on the use of proximity sensors and cameras when reversing.

A significant percentage of collisions involving statutory ambulance service vehicles occur while carrying out low-speed manoeuvres, especially those involving reversing.

Many, if not all, of these incidents could be avoided if basic standard procedures were diligently put into practice; often negligence or apathy have a major influence. A professional approach to the reversing task significantly reduces repair costs and vehicle downtime, as well as promoting safety and reducing the risk of personal injury.

This chapter outlines the best practice procedures that should be employed when carrying out low-speed manoeuvres, with an emphasis on the importance of teamwork.

Theory and Practice

The Highway Code sets out general rules and advice on reversing and manoeuvring for the benefit of all drivers. In addition, the following advice is given:

- Only turn the steering wheel while the vehicle is moving, thereby avoiding damage to the tyres, steering linkage and any power-assisted steering mechanisms.
- Utilise slow vehicle speed in conjunction with rapid hand movements on the steering wheel when manoeuvring in confined areas.
- In relation to speed, a good rule of thumb is no faster than walking pace.
- Turn the steering wheel in the direction of the next vehicle movement just before ending the previous movement.
- Keep the vehicle moving slowly, maintaining smooth speed control by coordinating the clutch and accelerator in manual vehicles, or by using the footbrake in automatic vehicles.
- Carefully observe the front of the vehicle as it swings left or right while carrying out reversing turns.
- Avoid over-revving the engine, remembering that engine tick over may be sufficient on level ground.

The Importance of Teamwork

Very few, if any, reversing collisions occur when a banksman is assisting the driver from the correct position outside the vehicle. This is the correct procedure.

This vantage point should always be at the rear nearside (unless there are unusual circumstances that make this unsafe or impractical) as this is the point furthest away from the driver. The banksman should stand at a safe distance from the rear of the vehicle, positioned for safety and in full view of driver.

Reverse audible warning signals are fitted for safety. Some makes of vehicle allow these audible alarms to be turned off so as not to cause disturbance at night. Consideration must be given to the safety of those around you (and whether a banksman is being used) if you are turning these warnings off.

With the driver in the driving seat and the banksman at the rear nearside, responsibilities are shared as follows.

The driver is responsible for:

- Making sure that the banksman can be clearly seen in the nearside mirror before commencing the manoeuvre
- Controlling the speed of the vehicle
- Bringing the vehicle to an immediate halt if the banksman disappears from view
- Ensuring that safety is maintained at the front and offside of the vehicle
- Ensuring any audible reverse warnings fitted are utilised
- Ensuring that the front nearside window is down to assist in hearing instructions.

The banksman is responsible for:

- Taking up a position at the rear nearside of the vehicle, in a position where they can be seen in the driver's nearside mirror
- Ensuring that their signals remain visible in the driver's nearside mirror by adjusting their position as the vehicle moves
- Ensuring safety at the rear and nearside of the vehicle, as well as roof clearance
- Ensuring that any audible reversing alarms fitted to the vehicle are operating correctly
- Ensuring that they use the appropriate signals and, if required, verbal instructions
- Maintaining concentration on the task
- Wearing suitable personal protective equipment as directed by service policy – this ensures that they are clearly visible to the driver.

Keeping the Banksman in View

It is vital that the attendant remains in the driver's view at all times. In the event of the banksman no longer being visible to the driver, the vehicle must be brought to an immediate standstill.

Prior to any manoeuvre, the driver and banksman must discuss and agree an appropriate course of action. It is important that standard, recognisable hand and arm signals are used (shown in Figure 4.1). These can be augmented by verbal instructions – opening both windows will facilitate this. The terminology should be clear and the use of the word 'stop' is advised to reinforce the equivalent arm or hand signal.

If the major hazard is to the rear of the nearside, the driver should concentrate on following the banksman's signals, with regular glances to the front of the vehicle and offside mirror to ensure safety. If the major hazard is to the front or offside, the driver should concentrate on these areas, with regular glances in the nearside mirror to ensure safety.

The banksman must not stand in a position directly between a moving vehicle and a stationary or solid object, such as a wall or another vehicle. Where it is not viable or it is impractical for the banksman to take up a position at the rear nearside, the best alternative should be adopted. Extra care should be taken in these circumstances.

Particular care should also be taken if a banksman is not on hand to assist or if working alone. Consideration should be given to obtaining assistance from a responsible person where available; if no other person is available the driver should consider exiting the vehicle to safely check their surroundings. The driver has full responsibility for the safety of the manoeuvre in these circumstances.

Limitations of Technology

Drivers should not totally rely on the technology of reversing sensors or rearward facing cameras as they often provide a distorted view or inaccurate feedback. These devices should only be regarded as an aid to the driver.

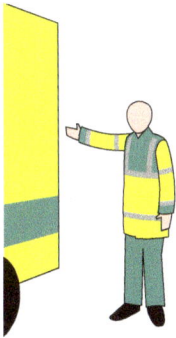

Banksman wants the driver to move to the right.

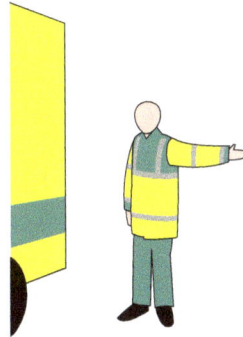

Banksman wants the driver to move to the left.

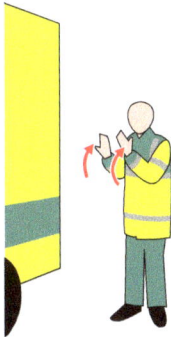

Banksman wants the driver to move rearwards in a straight line: the arms should be kept moving until another instruction is required.

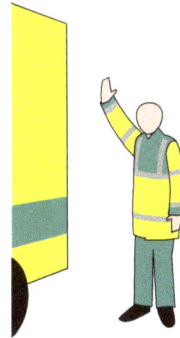

Banksman wants the driver to stop (both hands could be raised to give a clearer indication).

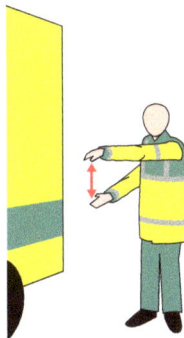

Banksman providing a visual reference of the gap remaining. Ensure arms are visible in the mirror and not obstructed by the body of the vehicle.

FIGURE 4.1 • Banksman using arm and hand signals.

? KNOWLEDGE RECAP

1   Why shouldn't the steering wheel be turned when the vehicle is stationary?
2   What is the best position for an assisting banksman to stand in when a reversing manoeuvre is being carried out?
3   What action should be taken if an assisting banksman disappears from the driver's view while reversing?
4   What precautions should be taken when reversing if a banksman is not present or available?

CHAPTER 5

Fuel-Efficient Driving

LEARNING OUTCOMES

By the end of this chapter you should:

- Understand what fuel-efficient driving means.
- Know the techniques that can be used to drive in a more environmentally friendly and economical way when not employing emergency response driving procedures.

While it is accepted that the nature of emergency response driving is not always conducive to fuel-efficiency due to the driving principles and systems engaged, there are many occasions when ambulance service vehicles drive under normal conditions and, therefore, every effort should be made to help to reduce the carbon footprint and fuel costs of the ambulance service.

This chapter outlines the ways in which ambulance drivers can reduce their fuel consumption by driving in the most energy-efficient way when not driving under emergency response conditions.

Economical Driving

Driving in a way that gets the most out of the fuel in your vehicle not only cuts down on greenhouse gas emissions and other pollutants, it also reduces costs. When not driving under emergency response conditions, drivers of ambulance service vehicles have a responsibility to contribute positively to this.

The AA (2017) offers the following advice on economical driving:

- **Smooth and gentle:** drive smoothly, accelerate gently and read the road ahead to avoid braking unnecessarily. Decelerate smoothly by releasing the accelerator in time, leaving the car in gear.
- **Keep rolling:** stopping then starting again uses more fuel than rolling. Slow early for traffic lights or approaching a queue and you might not have to stop completely.
- **Change up earlier:** don't labour the engine but try changing up at an engine speed of around 2,000 rpm (diesel) or 2,500 (petrol). Since 2014 new car models have been fitted with a gear shift indicator to encourage use of the most efficient gear.
- **Use your air-conditioning wisely:** at low speeds, having the air-conditioning on increases fuel consumption but at higher speeds the effect is less noticeable. Try opening the windows around town and save the air-conditioning for high-speed driving. Don't leave it on all the time, but running it at least once a week helps keep the system in good condition.
- **Cut down on the electrics:** turn off your rear window heater, demister fan and headlights when you don't need them.
- **Stick to the limit:** going faster uses more fuel. Drive at 70 mph and you'll use up to 9 per cent more than at 60 mph and up to 15 per cent more than at 50 mph. Driving at 80 mph can use up to 25 per cent more fuel than at 70 mph.

Unless the vehicle is fitted with a stop/start system, don't switch off the engine to save fuel unless you expect not to have to move for more than three minutes, for example at a level crossing, and you know that your vehicle has a well charged battery. Vehicles with stop/start systems have advanced components to make sure that when the engine stops it will be able to restart again.

⑦ KNOWLEDGE RECAP

1 What does fuel-efficient driving mean?
2 What are the benefits of driving in a more fuel-efficient way?
3 Describe three techniques that can be used to drive in a more environmentally friendly way.

CHAPTER 6

Ambulance Vehicles and Characteristics

LEARNING OUTCOMES

By the end of this chapter you should:

- Understand a range of different ambulance vehicles and their advantages and limitations.
- Know which types of vehicles may require extra training or familiarisation.
- Understand the differences associated with driving electric vehicles and the added safety precautions for these type of vehicle.

Vehicles will handle differently depending on their size, weight, drive trains, power to weight ratio and any active safety systems fitted. Consideration should be given to your ability to drive these different types of vehicles. This will depend on factors such as, the category of licence you hold, your familiarisation with the size & type of vehicle and how often you drive them. Is the vehicle type new to you or does it incorporate new technologies such as regenerative braking? As the driver it is your responsibility to ensure you understand how the vehicle controls and safety systems work, and how it will handle in different situations.

Ambulances

Ambulances now come in various designs, shapes and sizes. Whilst many require a C1 licence to drive, others can be driven on a conventional car licence. It is important to recognise that even those that do not require a C1 licence to drive, will handle very differently to a car. Weight, length and centre of gravity will all be vastly different to a car. This will affect the handling characteristics such as acceleration, cornering abilities and braking distances.

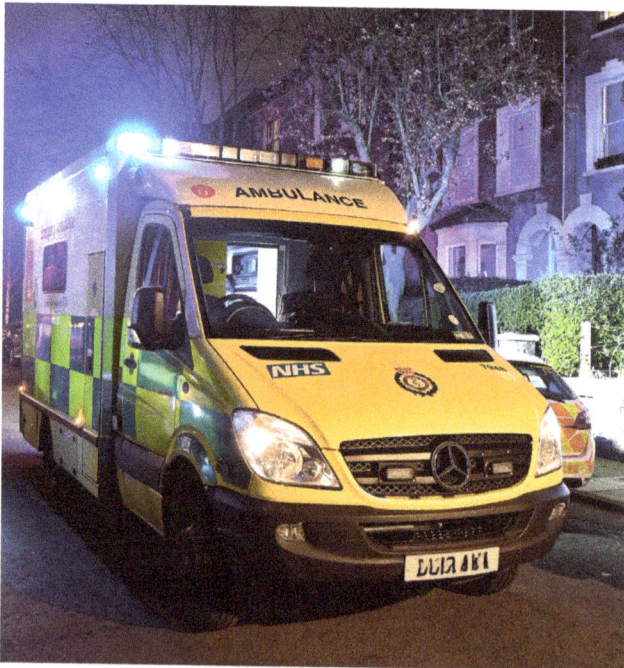

FIGURE 6.1 • Ambulance.

Being higher, they may be adversely affected by cross winds. Ambulances have space to carry a full range of equipment plus patients and crew. Consideration should be given to the difference in weight distribution when fully laden with patients, family members and extra crew such as critical care support staff.

Ambulances generally require increased servicing and maintenance schedules and are generally more expensive to purchase and run than other vehicles. Most ambulances are required to comply with the lower speed limits associated with goods vehicles.

Ambulance Response Cars

Due to the fact that cars are smaller and lighter than patient carrying ambulances, they are harder to see when approaching hazards and offer less view of the road ahead than from the raised position in an ambulance. Cars have a lower centre of gravity and so may offer improved stability when negotiating hazards. They are capable of accelerating quicker than an ambulance due to their power to weight ratio, however, with increased speed comes increased risk. Cars do not usually require an extra category of licence to drive and may be more fuel efficient than ambulances but have limited capacity to carry equipment, patients, and crew.

Unmarked Ambulance Response Vehicles

All of the considerations listed for the ambulance response vehicles above will apply equally to unmarked vehicles, with the added risk of being less visible due to lack of reflective markings and roof lights. Extra caution should be used when responding in unmarked vehicles and more time should be given for other road users to see you and acknowledge your presence, especially on the approach to fixed hazards such as roundabouts. Consideration should be given to extra training for the use of unmarked vehicles on response.

Motorcycles

Motorcycles are smaller and have a higher power to weight ratio than cars and ambulances. This gives them the ability to negotiate heavy traffic more easily, but with this comes an increased vulnerability for the rider. They are less visible due to their size and reduced reflective markings and lights when compared to an ambulance or car, and offer the rider less protection in the event of a collision. Other road users are less likely to see motorcycles and may not react appropriately or in enough time. Motorcycles may be able to access confined spaces and may be easier to park in congested areas. Motorcycles do not have the stability of four-wheeled vehicles and may not be able to operate in extremes of weather. Motorcycles require separate driving licence categories and additional specialist training to drive on response. Specialist, individual, PPE such as protective/reflective clothing will be required to ride motorcycles. While some of the principles and philosophies covered in this handbook can be applied universally to driving as well as riding motorcycles, response training for motorcycles is beyond the scope of this handbook.

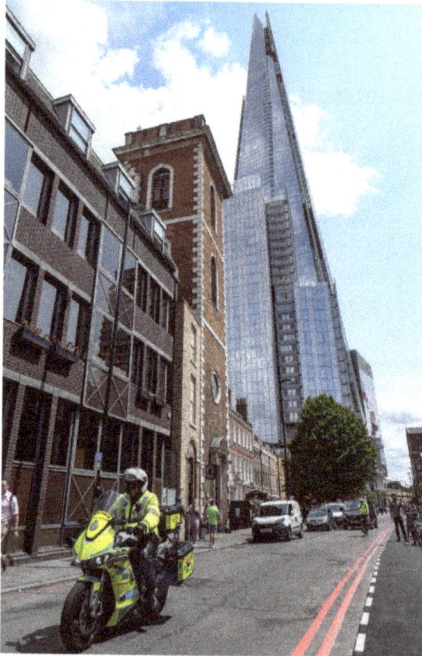

FIGURE 6.2 • Motorcycle.

LGVs

Some specialist teams or departments may have larger vehicles as part of their fleet, such as Specialist Operations Resilience Teams (SORT) or Hazardous Area Response Teams (HART). Whilst many of these can be driven on a C1 driving licence (up to 7.5T in weight), the handling characteristics can be very different to a conventional ambulance. The main considerations with larger vehicles are likely to be its weight, width, length and height. This will influence the distance that is required to emerge into the flow of traffic, the distance required to overtake another road user, the size of the gap required to manoeuvre around obstacles and the overall stopping distance. The driver will need to consider the vehicles capabilities when ascending or descending steep inclines. Often larger vehicles will be air braked and may have additional retarder or exhaust brakes. The vehicle may be fitted with a tail lift that requires isolation or other specialist equipment. Consideration must be given to how the vehicle is loaded and how the load is secured. Extra training should be undertaken prior to using such vehicles.

Bicycles

With the increase in low traffic neighbourhoods (LTNs), more NHS services are employing the use of bicycles in urban areas, or at events to be able to reach patients more effectively. Cycles are agile and can manoeuvre through pedestrianised areas with ease, as well as having less impact on the environment and reduced fuel costs. Cycles are only able to transport a limited amount of equipment and one crew. They are less visible in traffic and even with individual personal protective/reflective clothing, the rider is more vulnerable in a collision than in a vehicle.

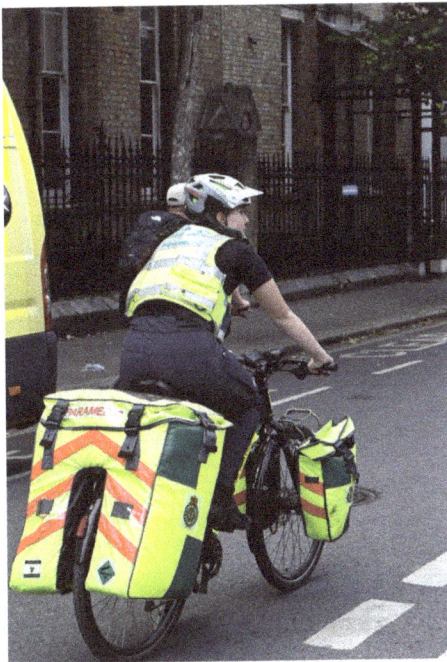

FIGURE 6.3 • Bicycle.

Electric Vehicles (EVs)

Electric vehicles function in a similar way to automatic vehicles when driving, with only forward/reverse gears and no clutch. Care should be taken as there may be no engine noise whilst the vehicle is switched on. Electric vehicle motors deliver instant power, and caution must therefore be taken in driving these vehicles, especially in adverse weather conditions or in 'sports' mode. Without engine noise drivers may be less likely to notice increased speed. Familiarisation training may be required.

Drivers should be fully conversant with the driving mileage 'range' of the vehicle which may be reduced when used for emergency response. Drivers should understand how to charge the vehicle either at station or using public chargers. Electric vehicles should never be charged using coiled extension leads or temporary plug sockets due to fire risk.

Regenerative braking uses kinetic energy to recharge the battery. This may help to increase driving range, however it will mean the vehicle slowing down more during deceleration, so the driver should be prepared for this and build it into their driving plan.

Hybrid electric vehicles utilise electric motors and internal combustion engines. The vehicle will swap from one power source to the other without any input from the driver.

Electric Vehicle Safety

EVs are designed to isolate the high voltage electrical system. However, some extra precautions should be taken when dealing with collisions or incidents involving electric vehicles as the lithium-ion battery cells may have been damaged.

- Damaged battery cells may appear to emit white or black steam or smoke. However, this is likely to be a toxic vapour cloud and should be avoided. Lithium battery fumes, especially those released during fires or thermal runaway, are hazardous and can contain toxic substances like hydrogen fluoride and carbon monoxide, posing risks of respiratory problems, skin irritation, and even poisoning.

- If hissing or popping noises are heard from damaged battery cells do not approach. Damaged battery cells can emit very long hot flames and may even explode without fire and without warning.

- EVs, like automatic vehicles, may still move without warning or driver input if still in gear. If safe to do so, power the vehicle off first.

- ORANGE cables connect the high voltage system. Do not touch these cables if exposed. Ensure these cables are not touching any extraneous conducting materials, such as street furniture, before approaching.

- If the vehicle has overturned or sustained high levels of damage, avoid touching or moving the vehicle, especially the underside, until the fire and rescue service have assessed and cleared it.

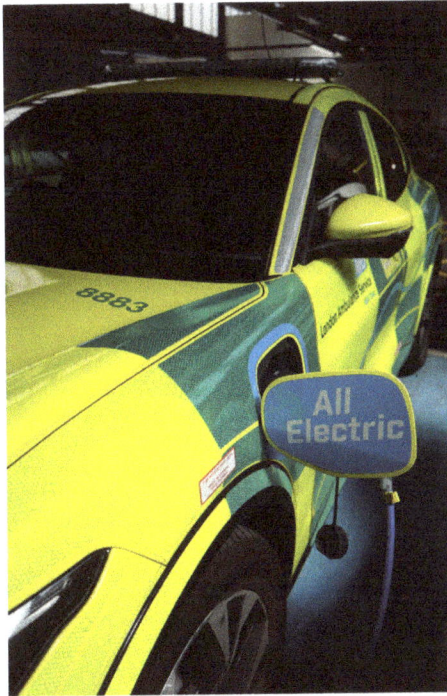

FIGURE 6.4 • Electric vehicle.

4x4 and Other Drive Trains

Specialist teams or those who require off road capability may employ 4x4 or all-terrain vehicles within their fleet. These vehicles may provide better traction on slippery or loose surfaces and in inclement weather. They may be used to convey equipment or patients to or from remote areas that other vehicles would struggle to reach. These vehicles may incur increased costs to purchase and maintain and may require extra training in order to make full use of the added features. Whilst 4x4 systems can provide added traction and stability, they should never be used as a substitute for an effective driving plan or as an excuse for poor driving techniques.

In all types of vehicles, you must drive to the prevailing hazards and conditions, not to the speed of the vehicle. The vehicle should always be driven within its own and the drivers' limitations for the prevailing conditions.

(?) KNOWLEDGE RECAP

1 What vehicle features will determine how it handles when driven?
2 Name two benefits of an ambulance response car?
3 Name two limitations of an ambulance motorcycle?
4 State one safety precaution when dealing with an incident involving an electric vehicle?

CHAPTER **7**

Automatic Gearboxes

LEARNING OUTCOMES

By the end of this chapter you should:

- Understand the functionality of the selector lever options.
- Know the principles of how and when to manually select lock down, sport or manual modes within the gearbox special programmes.
- Recognise the important characteristics of automatic gearboxes.
- Understand the terms 'creep', 'run on' and 'lock down'.
- Understand how to get the most out of an automatic transmission when driving an emergency response vehicle.

Many ambulance vehicles are fitted with an automatic transmission – these systems replace the need for a conventional clutch and gearbox so that the driver no longer has to shift gears manually. It is important that adequate training is received in their use in order for you to drive the vehicles correctly and safely.

As automatic gearboxes are becoming more common, it is essential that you know how to make the best use of them. This chapter outlines the general principles of automatic gearboxes – understanding them will enable you to make correct decisions, based on accurate driving plans with due consideration to the presence of various hazards and the performance of the vehicle.

Selector Lever Options

The selector lever is normally mounted on the dashboard, but it is sometimes on the floor or steering column, an example of which can be seen in Figure 7.1. Some vehicles have paddles or push-button mechanisms, so you should ensure through your PDC, and by reading the vehicle handbook, that you are familiar with the vehicle's selector lever and automatic gearbox controls.

An illuminated indicator panel, usually contained within LCD display on the dashboard, provides visual confirmation of the selector position currently engaged.

There are variations to the location of controls in automatic vehicles, but the function and principles remain the same.

The basic selector lever positions are explained below.

P (park)

'Park' should be selected when the vehicle is parked, before the engine is switched off. A check should be made that the selector is in this position before attempting to start the engine. To further ensure safety, the footbrake should be depressed while starting the engine.

Never move the lever to the 'P' position while the vehicle is in motion.

R (reverse)

'Reverse' is usually located next to 'Park' in the selector mechanism sequence. It is normally a requirement of the system that the footbrake is depressed when moving the selector from 'P' to 'R', or when moving from 'P' through 'R' to get to another selector option. The vehicle may begin to move backwards the instant the selector is moved into 'R', unless the brakes are applied.

N (neutral)

No power is transmitted from the engine to the drive wheels when in neutral. It should be selected when the vehicle needs to be towed after a breakdown or accident. It should not be selected when making temporary stops in traffic. You should consult the vehicle manual before towing or allowing the vehicle to be towed, as some systems may be damaged when the lever is left in 'N' and the vehicle's wheels are moving.

D (drive)

'Drive' is the regular operational mode to use when driving an automatic vehicle under normal driving conditions. It allows the transmission to make automatic adjustments according to your speed, engine loading and accelerator position. As the accelerator is depressed, and the vehicle gathers speed, sensors detect the optimum time to change up to the next highest gear. The change is made automatically, without the intervention of the driver. Harsh acceleration can result in jerky changes, while smooth and gradual increases in speed may make changes imperceptible to patients and other passengers.

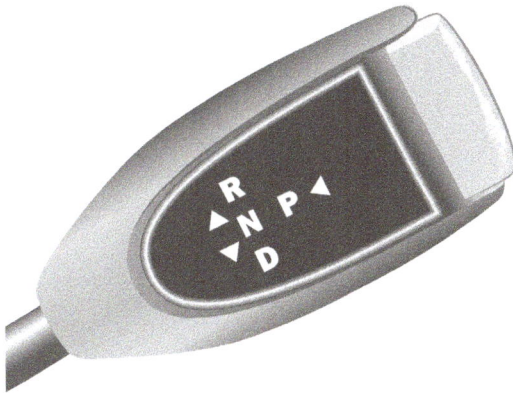

FIGURE 7.1 • An example of the positions of the selector lever:
- P: Park – prevents the vehicle from rolling away when stopped
- R: Reverse – only engage reverse gear when the vehicle is stationary
- N: Neutral – no power is transmitted from the engine to the drive wheels
- D: Drive – automatic drive uses all forward gears and a configuration for manual selection, or a plus and minus sign for upward and downward manual changes.

Driving Styles

Many modern automatic gearboxes adjust to the driver's driving style, holding a gear for longer and delaying an upshift when accelerating quickly, while changing up earlier when applying gentle acceleration.

Use of neutral

Remember that there is no need to move the gear lever into 'Neutral' when stationary in traffic, even for many minutes. No wear is taking place; in fact, more wear will take place if you put it into 'Neutral' then back into 'Drive' when you are ready to move off. You may find additional information on this in the vehicle handbook. Most gearboxes will automatically select first gear when your vehicle stops in anticipation of your next movement.

Safety warning

It is vitally important to remember that automatics do not have a clutch pedal. Depressing the footbrake with the left foot, in the mistaken belief that this is the clutch, can have disastrous consequences – particularly if the vehicle is being driven at speed or being followed too closely by another road user.

Automatics should always be left in 'Park' (P) when not being driven. When carrying out a pre-driving check, 'selector in P' should be substituted for 'gear lever in neutral'.

Manual Gear Select

In many instances the selector lever can remain in 'D' for ordinary driving. During response driving, or in situations where additional control is required, then an advantage may be gained by selecting one of the vehicle's special programmes. Each vehicle manufacturer may have different systems, but generally they fall into the following categories – note a vehicle may be fitted with more than one of the options below:

- Lock down (or shift restrictions)
- Sport
- Manual selection.

Lock Down (or Shift Restrictions)

This is an effective means of controlling an automatic gearbox while descending steep gradients, overtaking or negotiating a corner or roundabout to ensure vehicle stability. The number of lock down options (or restrictions) varies and depends on how many gears the vehicle has. The number of lock down options will always be less than the total number of gears present: a five-speed gearbox may have four lock down options, while a vehicle with four gears may have three.

Alternative lock down positions may be used to control the vehicle like a manual clutchless vehicle. In all cases, the maximum upshift will be represented by the lock down position selected, for example if lock down position 4 has been selected then the vehicle will utilise all gears up to and including the fourth gear, but will not go into fifth or sixth gear.

You might choose to lock down a lower gear in a built-up area, where there are a number of hazards, to improve control through the accelerator. However, the gear you select should always be appropriate for your circumstances. In a five-speed automatic gearbox, third gear may be most suitable for urban driving while fourth may be a better and more flexible choice for rural roads.

It is essential to remember to move the selector back to 'Drive' when the need to utilise lock down has passed. Driving the vehicle for a prolonged period in a lock down option can overheat the automatic transmission fluid and cause damage to the transmission system.

Sport Mode

The sport setting is more often fitted to car and 4x4-type vehicles, rather than commercial vehicles. By selecting this option the gearbox will hold lower gears for longer, allowing for brisker acceleration as the gearbox may not need to change down a gear in order to accelerate at maximum power.

Sport mode may also disengage or change other vehicle systems, such as the electronic stability programme (ESP), antilock brake system (ABS) or start–stop technology and as such you should familiarise yourself with the vehicle's set-up prior to use.

Manual Selection

Some vehicles may be fitted with a manual selection of the gears through the selected lever or steering wheel-mounted paddles or buttons. These systems allow the driver to select the gear as though they were driving a manual vehicle, but without the need for a clutch. In these circumstances, the gears can be selected according to your needs and your driving plan. For example, on the approach to a steep downhill section, a lower gear could be selected prior to descent. Likewise, you may choose to secure a lower gear prior to negotiating a corner.

In all cases, moving the selector lever (or paddles) between modes is best done when under light acceleration. Care must be taken to ensure that the selector is moved the correct number of steps to reach the desired position. The gear selected must be appropriate for the speed that you are travelling at – most modern systems will override your lever selection if the engine revs or speed are too high.

Practice is essential to allow accuracy when attention cannot be diverted from the road ahead to check the indicator panel.

> ### ⓘ REMEMBER
>
> With both automatic and manual gearboxes, you must be travelling at the correct speed for the gear that you want to select manually. Secondary braking should be avoided.

Important Characteristics of Automatic Gearboxes

Creep

If any selector position other than 'P' or 'N' is selected, and the footbrake or handbrake are not applied, then the vehicle will tend to creep forward or backward at low speed, even when pressure is not applied to the accelerator pedal.

The rate of creep varies in response to the force of gravity. Consequently, creep will be greater on a downhill slope than an uphill slope. Creep can, and must, be controlled by using the footbrake. It is particularly useful when manoeuvring at low speeds or in slow moving traffic.

Creep may not hold a vehicle still on a steep hill. In such cases the handbrake should be used.

Run On

Deceleration in a vehicle fitted with manual transmission is relatively straightforward – releasing pressure on the accelerator pedal slows the engine and deceleration is achieved by means of engine compression. This is especially effective in lower gears. This is not the case in an automatic vehicle when driving with the selector set in the 'D' position. Releasing pressure on the accelerator will not result in a change down to a lower gear, nor is engine compression apparent.

This is referred to as 'run on' and provides a driving sensation similar to 'coasting'. If the vehicle is travelling uphill, gravity will slow it down. If the vehicle is travelling downhill, however, the combined effects of run on and gravity will result in a progressive increase in speed. Steep downward slopes can produce an alarming sensation of losing control as gravity takes over and vehicle speed rises sharply.

The timely and judicious use of lock down or a manual selection will effectively prevent this potentially dangerous circumstance. When driving on level stretches of road, early relaxation of pressure on the accelerator will facilitate more effcient acceleration sense.

Kick Down

This is a useful safety feature that should only be used when there is actual or potential danger. It provides short-term bursts of maximum acceleration, to escape from hazardous circumstances, without the need to move the selector lever.

Apply the accelerator pedal downwards rapidly to the furthest limit of its travel. After a very brief interval the transmission will change down to the next lowest gear and rapid acceleration will ensue. Holding the pedal down may result in a further subsequent change down and yet more acceleration. You then have a mechanism to escape from danger by using maximum acceleration when this is appropriate. Relaxing pressure on the accelerator results in loss of acceleration and a change back up to a higher gear.

Care must be taken when using kick down. Plan and look well ahead to ensure that the vehicle is not powered out of one dangerous situation and into another.

ⓘ KEY TERMS

Creep – the tendency of an automatic vehicle to creep forwards or backwards at low speed, even when pressure is not applied to the accelerator.

Run on – the tendency of an automatic vehicle not to reduce speed when pressure is no longer applied to the accelerator; the vehicle may even gain speed if travelling downhill.

Kick down – a feature of automatic vehicles that allows you to accelerate suddenly, overriding the automatic selection of gears.

Electric and Hybrid Vehicles

Although most electric and hybrid vehicles are fitted with automatic gearboxes they do not all have the same features mentioned here.

For example, they may not 'run on' when the accelerator is released, due to energy recuperation. This may mean that you need additional training, guidance or instruction on operating them. In all cases you should ensure through a pre-driving check that you are familiar with their controls, and ensure that you have read the vehicle handbook.

Automatic Vehicles in Emergency Response Driving

Although some ambulance services advocate a more direct manual use of automatic gearboxes, particularly in response situations, the lock down, sport or manual override facility should not be used excessively. If you do not require a greater degree of flexibility or maximum performance from the vehicle, you should consider carefully whether it is really necessary.

While it is impossible to provide gear selection guidance for all eventualities, the following advice is intended to provide some general guidance in some common sets of circumstances.

- **Control over speed:** when you need more control over acceleration – for example in response to a particular hazard, when overtaking or approaching an area of uncertainty – manually selecting a particular gear will prevent the gearbox from changing up automatically, providing more flexibility to control speed. Once the need for this flexibility has passed, however, the 'D' option should be considered.

- **Stopping:** apply the footbrake before moving the selector lever when the vehicle is stationary. Set the parking brake, as many automatic vehicles will creep and some have a tendency to lurch. Leave the selector in 'D' when stopped in traffic, at junctions and at traffic lights. There is no need to move into neutral.

- **At roundabouts:** engage the appropriate gear in lock down, sport or manual mode on the approach to the hazard to provide greater vehicle stability.

- **On bends:** gentle bends can normally be negotiated in 'D'. For a series of bends, however, manually select a suitable gear before the first bend. On exiting that bend, when the accelerator is eased in preparation for the next bend, the vehicle will not automatically change up. This provides the benefit of engine braking, which gives better control.

- **Overtaking:** when overtaking you can choose to either manually select a lower gear or use the 'kick down' function. If you need to accelerate then decelerate rapidly to fit into a gap, manually selecting a lower gear before the start of the manoeuvre may be beneficial.

- **Steep hills:** when descending steep hills in 'D', automatic vehicles have a tendency to change into a higher gear, which can necessitate the need for excessive braking. This can induce 'brake fade' – a reduction in stopping power after sustained or repeated braking. This can be overcome by manually locking or changing down to a low ratio gear, which will then provide compression braking to enhance vehicle braking. Similarly, when ascending steep hills, changing or locking a ratio manually can provide better control.

Dos and Don'ts for Automatic Vehicles

- Never select 'P' while the vehicle is in motion. It will cause major damage or an accident by locking the transmission.
- Only engage reverse gear when the vehicle is stationary, otherwise the transmission could be damaged.
- Ensure that the footbrake is on before engaging either 'D' or 'R' from stationary.
- Do not engage 'D' or 'R' with a high-revving engine.

Knowing When to Switch to Manual – and When Not To

In commercial vehicles, when the engine is under strain, manually selecting a gear can be useful in circumstances when the gear box is continually changing up and down between two gears. This can also reduce wear on the gearbox.

It is not always necessary to select a lower gear manually for a hazard as you might do when driving a manual vehicle. Modern automatic gearboxes are designed to select the correct ratio for the speed and throttle setting. However, manual selection should be considered if this would offer better stability for the vehicle in respect of the circumstances encountered at the time.

Realistically, it is not possible to determine all the occasions when 'D' would be a better choice than switching to manual gears. You must execute accurate judgement and consider your driving plans to judge which is most appropriate. Avoid making unnecessary or excessive use of the manual hold position – you should return to 'D' when the need has passed.

Automatics can make driving appear easier by removing the need to make recurring changes of gear while concentrating on maintaining smooth clutch control. Diligent application of the above principles will ensure that you get the best from your vehicle while maintaining full control without compromising safety margins.

> ### ⓘ KEY TERMS
>
> **Brake fade** – a reduction in stopping power after sustained or repeated braking.

(?) KNOWLEDGE RECAP

1   Name the four basic gear selector positions in an automatic vehicle.
2   What would happen if the gear lever was moved into the 'P' (Park) position while the vehicle was in motion?
3   In what circumstances would you select the 'N' (Neutral) position?
4   Why should you always consider moving the gear selector back to 'D' (Drive) after a period of lock down, manual or sport mode operation?
5   What is 'creep' and how is it best controlled?
6   Releasing pressure on the accelerator of a manual vehicle usually results in the vehicle slowing down. Why is this not always the case for automatic vehicles?

CHAPTER 8

Vehicle Operating and Safety Systems

LEARNING OUTCOMES

By the end of this chapter you should:

- Be able to identify the various types of braking and brake assist systems.
- Recognise the various dashboard warning lamps that indicate brake system malfunctions.
- Understand the purpose of retarder systems.
- Understand the various vehicle stability, traction control, cruise control and hill hold features.
- Know how to operate the run lock system.
- Demonstrate how to connect electrical charge support systems to the vehicle and isolate the batteries.
- Correctly operate all emergency lighting controls.
- Identify the various electrical emergency warning malfunction lights and take the appropriate action.

The NHS ambulance service has evolved considerably over the years, from operating a fleet of vehicles specifically designed for the purpose of conveying patients, to a range of bespoke vehicles including response cars, resilience vehicles, motorcycles and specialist vehicles.

In this chapter we consider some of the vehicle operating systems and safety features that you are likely to encounter when driving ambulance vehicles. These include the key fob, braking and stability systems, electrical control systems, emergency warning equipment (EWE) controls and dashboard warning lights.

Brake Systems

Most modern ambulance vehicles offer a number of safety systems to assist with vehicle braking. Figure 8.1 provides an example of typical dashboard warning lights that identify some of these systems. Note that this is intended to provide an example and that there are other similar systems in operation. You will be able to find details of the specific dashboard warning lights in the manual for the vehicle.

Emergency Brake Assist

Emergency brake assist (EBA) is designed to operate during emergency braking situations. When the brake pedal is depressed quickly, the EBA automatically increases the brake pressure, reducing the stopping distance. The system interprets braking behaviour by assessing the rate at which the brake pedal is activated and initiates full braking.

If the EBA malfunctions or fails, the vehicle will still have its full brake effect but the stopping distance may increase.

Antilock Brake System

When the antilock brake system (ABS) is activated, this enables you to steer and brake without the wheels locking during harsh braking. A pulsating of the brake pedal will be experienced. ABS is designed to be the technical equivalent to 'cadence braking'. The ABS light may illuminate for a short period of time to warn you that the system has been triggered. If this light stays illuminated, there is a fault with the system and the vehicle will need to be checked by a mechanic.

Electronic Brake Force Distribution

Electronic brake force distribution (EBD) monitors and controls the brake pressure placed upon the wheels to improve vehicle handling while braking.

It will detect which wheel has more or less grip and will vary the braking force to the wheels to reduce the chance of skidding.

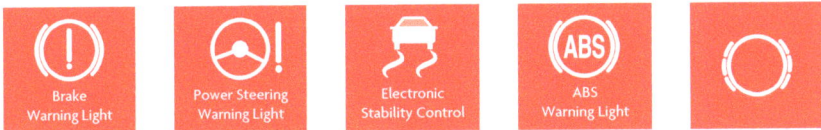

FIGURE 8.1 • Warning lights showing:
- Electronic brakeforce distribution system malfunction
- Electric power steering fault malfunction
- Electronic stability control (ESC) system failure
- ABS
- Brake pads/linings worn.

Retarders

Retarders are often fitted to large vehicles – they assist the braking systems by helping to slow the vehicle down, at any speed, while ensuring a smooth ride. The system is often fully automatic and the control system is normally activated by the action of the driver depressing the brake pedal, requiring no additional driver input and no special training.

Most modern retarders fitted to ambulance vehicles are electromagnetic. They reduce the workload of the brakes and eliminate the risks associated with the brakes overheating. Electromagnetic retarders slow down the rotating driveshaft using electromagnetic forces, without the need for any friction.

The retarder system reaction time is virtually instantaneous. This makes for optimum compatibility with ABS. Application of the footbrake operates the circuits in the control box, which close, and energise the retarder, which applies the 'friction-free' braking torque to the rear wheels, slowing the vehicle down. In most vehicles there is a red 'R' warning light that will illuminate during this function; it is normally situated close to the instrument panel (see Figure 8.2).

You should ensure that you know what type of system is fitted to your vehicle and follow any manufacturer-specific instructions.

Retarder systems have, in some instances, been shown to automatically absorb more than 80 per cent of braking applications. This helps in keeping brake temperatures low. High brake temperatures lead to brake fade and wear, increased maintenance costs and increased vehicle downtime.

Retarder systems can also help reduce overall stopping distances, provided that tyre adhesion is maintained, giving obvious benefits to the crew, patients and other road users.

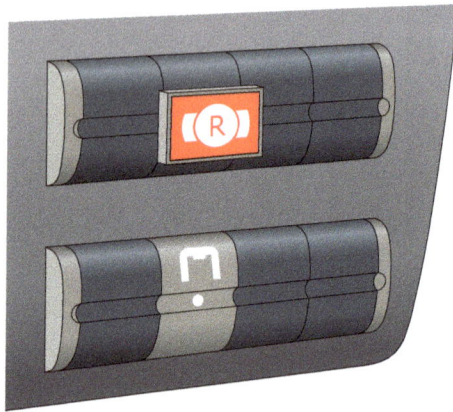

FIGURE 8.2 • The red 'R' warning light.

Another benefit is that the system slows the vehicle via the rear axle and, when braking, this contributes to keeping the vehicle level, eliminating most of the front-end 'dipping'. This provides a considerable improvement in vehicle stability when braking, both in a straight line and when cornering, with reduced 'roll' of the vehicle and a greater sense of confidence in the overall handling.

Traction Control Systems

Most modern vehicles are equipped with various stability systems that are designed to assist with maximising traction while the vehicle is in motion. While traction control was once a standalone safety feature, there are now a number of different systems and it is important you are aware of what is fitted to the vehicles you are driving. Some of the systems you may come across are explained below.

Acceleration Skid Control or Anti-Slip Regulator

Skid control or anti-slip mechanisms are a form of traction control. Acceleration skid control (ASC), also known as an anti-slip regulator (ASR), transfers the power from the tyres to the road surface for a set period. This results in improved stability of the vehicle. ASR also assists when moving off and accelerating, especially on smooth or slippery surfaces. ASR works by applying brake effect to individual drive wheels and reducing the engine torque to prevent the drive wheels from spinning.

A warning light in the instrument cluster flashes when ASC/ASR is active. Although ASR can be switched off on most vehicles as it is a safety feature, it must not be deactivated during normal use.

Electronic Stability Control

The electronic stability control (ESC) is an evolution of traction control and works in a similar way to ASR. It is able to predict when the vehicle may under- or oversteer, which could result in the vehicle skidding. It works by recovering vehicle stability by braking individual wheels and reducing power output from the engine.

The system is valuable when driving on wet or slippery road surfaces where tyre grip is reduced. Similar to an ASR system, a warning light may flash when the system is active. It is important to understand that this system can't remove the risk of a collision – if the vehicle speed is excessive or inappropriate for the road conditions, ESP will not work. It is not possible to override the laws of physics!

Lane Departure Warning

A lane departure warning system uses a camera or infrared sensor to watch road markings and detect if the vehicle strays away from the lane it is travelling in. It then warns you with either a buzzer or vibration. More advanced systems will take corrective action and steer the vehicle back into the lane if the driver does not take the appropriate action. The system does not remove the need for you to concentrate.

Hill Hold Assist

The hill hold assist function is an electronic safety aid that prevents the car from rolling backwards when the brake pedal is released. The device holds the brakes on until the clutch has reached the friction point, then releases them, allowing for a hill start to be performed without the risk of the vehicle rolling backwards.

Most systems engage when the vehicle is stationary and the nose is sufficiently higher than the rear of the car and holds the hydraulic pressure on the brakes, keeping the brake pads pressed against the brake discs even when the foot is removed from the brake pedal. On pulling away the brake pressure is released when the clutch takes up the weight of the vehicle.

Some systems will also prevent the car from rolling forwards on a downhill slope. It is important you are familiar with the function of the system fitted to the vehicle you are driving as, although some will hold the car indefinitely once the system is in operation, some only operate for short periods of time once the foot brake is released.

Cruise Control

First introduced in the 1940s, cruise control is a system that can automatically control the speed of a vehicle, using a servomechanism (or in newer vehicles an electronic system) to control the throttle, maintaining a steady speed set by you. Usually there will be steering wheel mounted controls for setting and adjusting the speed of the vehicle. It can often be cancelled by pressing the brake or clutch pedal.

If your vehicle is fitted with cruise control it is important you are familiar with the controls prior to using it; instructions can be found in the owner's manual. Cruise control can help reduce driver fatigue and improve the fuel economy of the vehicle. It can also help with maintaining legal speed limits.

Some modern vehicles now have adaptive cruise control that can react to the distance between the vehicle and the rear of any traffic in front. This can then vary the speed of the vehicle to maintain a safe travelling distance. These systems can often apply gentle braking pressure to slow the vehicle and may even vary the speed of the vehicle to the legal speed limit using GPS and road data.

Cruise control is an aid designed to assist driving, but you are always responsible for the speed and braking of the vehicle. Cruise control should not be used in traffic where the speed may vary suddenly (such as urban driving), on slippery surfaces or where visibility is poor. It may also be unable to maintain the speed of the vehicle on downhill sections. Cruise control should not be used during emergency response driving.

Run Lock Systems

Emergency vehicles are often equipped with a run lock system, which allows you to remove the ignition key for security reasons while the engine continues to operate to maintain electrical charge. This is of particular importance in modern-day ambulance vehicles due to the extensive range of electrical equipment fitted, such as data systems, telecommunications, medical devices, heating and emergency warning lights.

In the event of an attempted theft of the vehicle, the engine would cut out if the vehicle was to be driven away without the keys in the ignition. You should follow your service's guidelines when using these systems to ensure compliance with policy and law.

Electrical and Emergency Lighting Control Systems

Due to the volume and variety of electrical equipment fitted to modern emergency ambulance vehicles and the subsequent power demand, especially while stationary, many vehicles are fitted with a number of batteries.

- **Link bar low power button:** the link bar low power button can be utilised if a battery drain is affecting engine ignition. Power is sourced from an auxiliary battery that should be sufficient to start the vehicle.

- **Electrical umbilical leads (shore lines):** while stationary and parked for prolonged periods, such as at ambulance stations, emergency vehicles should be connected to umbilical electrical charge leads where available. They ensure the batteries receive constant charge. Although the lead system is designed to automatically disconnect when the engine starts, confirmation of this must be established as part of the moving-off procedure.

- **Isolators:** most vehicles will also be equipped with isolation switches that can be used for emergency isolation, if required, or to preserve battery power when vehicles are parked for extensive periods.

Emergency Lighting Controls

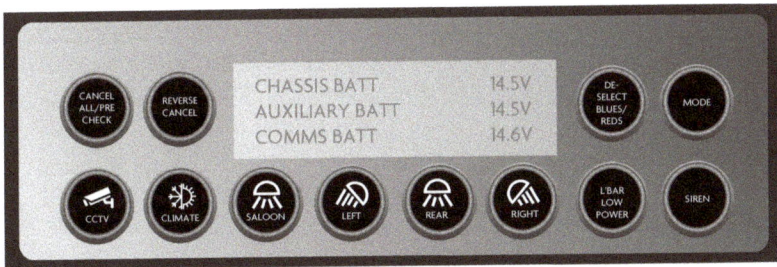

FIGURE 8.3 • Lighting controls.

Pre-Check Mode

This is a special feature button that can only be activated when the ignition and handbrake are both on. When pressed and held for five seconds it activates every function that can be visually inspected, individually and sequentially, in a predetermined order.

999 Mode

If this mode is selected, the appropriate emergency lighting is activated for response driving. It will also normally prepare the siren for activation using the horn button or foot switch.

Arrive Scene Mode

If 'arrive scene mode' is selected when the ignition is on, you can remove the ignition key and leave the engine running securely. Depending on the specification, the engine's speed may increase from idle. This will obviously not operate if the vehicle is in gear (or 'D' selected in an automatic).

This mode will also turn off the flashing headlights and switch on the rear red flashing lights (if fitted). Other blue lights will stay illuminated to maintain scene safety. If the handbrake is released the engine will stall.

Although modern ambulances have a significant power demand, it is important not to leave them idling for long periods of time just to preserve battery power. This has a negative impact on the environment, is not good for the engine and also causes noise pollution. Idling time should be kept to a minimum and where possible the vehicle should be connected to a shore line.

Arrive Hospital Mode

If the ignition is on when this mode is selected, the ignition security feature (run lock) will be activated, allowing you to remove the ignition key, but leave the engine running securely. This mode will also turn off any emergency warning systems that were active and turn on the saloon lights.

Siren Activation

The siren is activated by pressing the button on the control panel, where the sound, or tone, can normally be switched on or changed by pressing the vehicle horn or, where fitted, the foot switch. The siren can be deactivated by pressing the vehicle horn or foot switch twice, or by pressing the button on the control panel. Some vehicles may also be fitted with an auxiliary 'bull horn' operated from a separate switch on the dashboard.

The control panel may have numerous other functions, such as controlling internal saloon lighting, external scene lighting and operating auxiliary heating and air conditioning. It is your responsibility to be familiar with the controls for the vehicle you are driving.

System Failure

To reduce the risk of collisions, remember that if any of the icons below stay illuminated while on a journey, there may be a malfunction in one of the safety systems. You should drive with particular care and ensure that the fault is investigated as soon as possible by a mechanic.

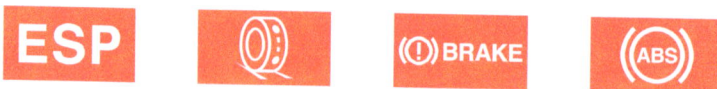

FIGURE 8.4 • Safety warning lights.

If any of the warning lights in the instrument cluster flash, you should proceed as follows:

- Do not deactivate any of the safety systems under normal circumstances.
- Depress the accelerator pedal only as far as necessary when pulling away.
- Adapt your driving style to suit the road and weather conditions, otherwise the vehicle could start to skid.

If any of the safety system warning lights are constantly lit when the engine is running, there may a malfunction or that system may be turned off. Check whether the system has been turned off and, if so, turn it back on. If the light does not go out, then the system has malfunctioned and the vehicle may reduce the engine power output. The fault needs to be investigated as soon as possible.

When driving a new vehicle for the first time it is important to check what safety systems are fitted to that specific model of vehicle and how they operate.

(?) KNOWLEDGE RECAP

1 Name three safety features that are normally found in emergency response vehicles to assist the braking system.
2 Describe what happens if the emergency brake assist (EBA) system malfunctions.
3 Describe how an electromagnetic retarder system works.
4 Why should high brake temperatures be avoided?
5 Describe how safety systems work and why they should not be deactivated under normal circumstances.
6 What is the purpose of a run lock system?
7 Why should emergency vehicles be connected to umbilical electrical charge leads (shore lines) when stationary or parked for prolonged periods at an ambulance station?

CHAPTER 9

Navigation

LEARNING OUTCOMES

By the end of this chapter you should:

- Understand how the satellite navigation in a modern ambulance works.
- Understand the importance of complying with road traffic law while using a sat nav.
- Be able to identify the components of a grid reference and how to find a location on a map using these.
- Understand how best to give directional instructions to a colleague who is driving.

Navigation is an important skill for ambulance staff. Whether using local knowledge, traditional map-reading skills or relying on satellite navigation, there is a need to be able to find your way to familiar locations such as local hospitals and ambulance stations, and to lesser-known locations such as patients' addresses and hospitals further afield. Staff need to be able to give clear and concise directional information to a colleague as well as interpret information given to them by others.

Satellite Navigation

Satellite navigation (or sat nav) is now commonplace and most people will be familiar with how to use it. Sat navs use global positioning system (GPS) signals to establish the current position of the vehicle and that, combined with a stored set of road maps, allows the system to plan a route from the current location to any selected destination. By constantly updating the vehicle's position using GPS, progress along the route can be plotted.

Many ambulance vehicles now have fixed sat navs that are part of a mobile data terminal. This means that the location of the vehicle can also be automatically communicated back to the control room. Such sat nav systems can often have the destination automatically populated by an incoming emergency from the control room, although they can usually be manually programmed as well.

Most sat nav systems will give visual prompts on a screen as well as voiced directions such as 'take the next right' or 'in 100 yards cross the roundabout, second exit'. The visual prompts are often in the form of a 2D or 3D map, with more detailed road layout schematics for junctions being approached.

It is safer to follow the verbal prompts rather than the visual ones, as this does not mean taking your eyes off the road – although a quick glance at a visual prompt may assist with negotiating complex junctions. Although these prompts will assist you with your journey, it is important to remember that you still need to comply with road traffic law.

The sat nav may not be aware of vehicle weight restrictions, temporary restrictions to access or changes to road layout, and it is up to the driver to interpret the information and act in accordance with road traffic law. The sat nav is an aid to your driving but is not in charge!

Dynamic Route Planning

Most sat nav systems have dynamic route planning, meaning that if you miss a turning or choose to take a different route, the route will be recalculated and updated accordingly.

To reduce distractions, new mobile data systems will automatically switch from job data to navigation. These include safety features such as voice activation and control to allow for hands-free interaction. Sat navs should not be programmed while driving, as this would mean taking your hands off the steering wheel and your eyes off the road. It is also important that the positioning of the sat nav does not block your view of the road, although it should be positioned so that it can easily be seen without the driver having to take their eyes off the road.

Maps

There may be times when you are unable to rely on the use of a sat nav to guide you on your journey. In these cases it is useful for you to be able to read a map. You cannot drive and read a map at the same time, but you may be in a situation where you have to read a map and convey directional instructions to a colleague.

For navigation in a vehicle, the best map to use is a road atlas. These tend to have a combination of national and local maps that vary in scale and detail. The large maps are useful for plotting travel over bigger distances, such as between towns and cities, whereas the more detailed local maps will be needed for identifying streets within a town.

To start with you need to be able to find your current location and your destination on the map. You may be able to do this using the index in the back of the atlas, which should give you a page number and a grid reference. In any grid reference (whether it uses letters or numbers or a mixture of both) the x-axis (horizontal) is shown first and the y-axis (vertical) is shown second. Plot the best route between the two locations – this might not be the shortest route as the crow flies but via main roads over a slightly longer distance.

Identifying Roads and Landmarks on a Map

Make sure that you are familiar with how different roads are represented on the map, for example motorways are often blue in colour and A roads often appear as a green line. Once you have set off, use landmarks on the map to assist in plotting progress against a route. It is also important to understand the scale of the map as this will help you know how far you are likely to have travelled against the overall distance of the journey. It may not look far on a map, but if the scale is small you may have travelled a long way.

It may help to follow the progress of the journey on the map with your finger; this way you are less likely to get lost. If you are providing directions to a colleague, it is important they are clear, concise and given at the most appropriate time. Do not give too many directions at once and make sure that your colleague has understood the instruction given.

When receiving directional instructions from a colleague, it is important to follow the same rules as when receiving prompts from a sat nav. You are still in charge of the vehicle and need to make sure that you comply with road traffic law at all times. If you are unsure of any instruction that your colleague has given, ask them to repeat it.

Whether you are using a modern sat nav system, or relying on the map-reading skills of a colleague while driving, it is important to remember that safe control of the vehicle is of paramount importance. The instructions being given, whether through visual or verbal prompts, should not distract you from concentrating on the road.

⑦ KNOWLEDGE RECAP

1 When reading a grid reference, is the first number or letter the x-axis or y-axis?
2 What does GPS stand for?
3 What limitations may sat navs have when using a larger or heavier vehicle?

CHAPTER 10

Legal Exemptions

LEARNING OUTCOMES

By the end of this chapter you should:

- Understand the legal exemptions available to drivers of ambulances when dealing with any category of patient.
- Understand the legal exemptions available to drivers of ambulances only while en route to an emergency.
- Be aware that contravening of any other road traffic law outside the exemptions provided by statute could render a driver liable to prosecution.

Drivers of ambulances may claim an exemption from certain road traffic legislation when justifiable and when the vehicle is being used for ambulance purposes. Provided:

- The observance of the law would be likely to hinder the use of the vehicle for the purpose for which it is being used.
- Nothing the driver does could be classed as being dangerous or careless.

This chapter offers advice and guidance in relation to the claiming of specific legal exemptions.

Claiming Legal Exemptions

It is essential that emergency response drivers are aware of the exemptions that apply to them and remember that there is still an overriding requirement to ensure the use of any exemption is safe and proportionate to the existing circumstances. The use of any exemption may have to be justified in a court of law.

The driver and the organisation are obliged, under the **Health and Safety at Work etc. Act 1974** and the **Road Safety Act 2006**, to afford, at all times, the maximum protection to other road users.

Prior to exercising any exemption derived from road traffic legislation you should ask yourself the following questions:

- Is the vehicle suitable? Any fault that results in the emergency equipment being defective could render the vehicle unsuitable.
- Does the nature of the call justify any exemption claimed? This could change during any journey.
- Can I justify the use of the vehicle's warning equipment? Can I justify not using the vehicle's warning equipment?
- What is the public perception of the actions I take? For example passing a school at high speed at 'going home' time.

The Vehicle Itself

Any fault that results in the emergency equipment being defective could mean that the vehicle is unsuitable. This includes:

- Fitting of audible warning instrument (siren or two-tone horns): Regulation 37(4) **Road Vehicles (Construction & Use) Regulations 1986**
- Use of reflective material on rear of vehicle: Regulation 11, **Road Vehicles Lighting Regulations 1989**

- Use of headlight flashing units: Regulation 13(2)(b), **Road Vehicles Lighting Regulations 1989**
- Use of flashing blue/red lighting equipment: Regulation 16, **Road Vehicles Lighting Regulations 1989**
- Side reflective materials: Part 2, Schedule 17, **Road Vehicles Lighting Regulations 1989**.

Road Traffic Law Exemptions That Apply When Dealing With Any Category of Patient

Parking Within the Controlled (Zig-zag) Area of a Pedestrian Crossing

Schedule 14, Part 1, Paragraph 14 (3)(c)(iii), **The Traffic Signs Regulations and General Directions 2016**

- Always ensure that you have the correct PPE when exiting the vehicle on 'fast' roads.
- Consider how your position may restrict the view of pedestrians using the crossing or of drivers approaching the crossing.
- Consider this to be a last resort – contemplate alternative options.
- Do not park across the crossing itself (the pedestrian crossing point).
- Consider positioning your vehicle on the exit side of the crossing.
- Consider requesting the assistance of police for traffic control.
- Consider use of hazard warning lights.
- Leaving a vehicle in a dangerous position is an offence and an exemption to this cannot be claimed.

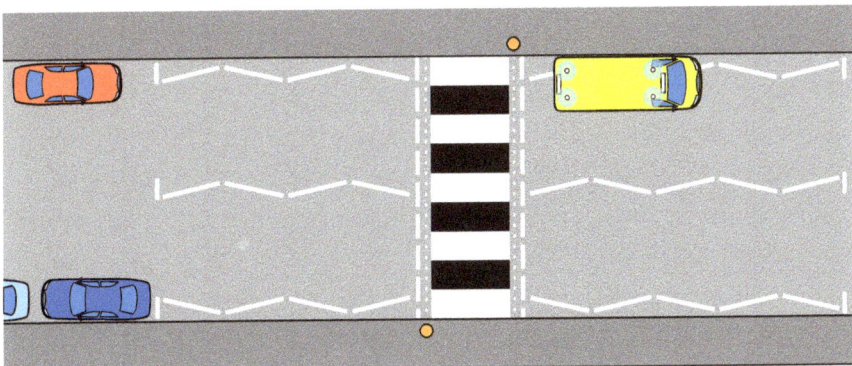

FIGURE 10.1 • Parking within the zig-zag area of a pedestrian crossing.

Parking Within Areas Controlled by Double White Lines

Schedule 9, Part 7, Paragraph 9(4)(iv), **Traffic Sign and General Directions 2016**

- Always ensure that you have the correct PPE when exiting the vehicle.
- Consider danger when boarding a patient on a stretcher.
- Keep time parked to a minimum.
- Consider use of hazard warning lights.
- Leaving a vehicle in a dangerous position is an offence and an exemption to this cannot be claimed.

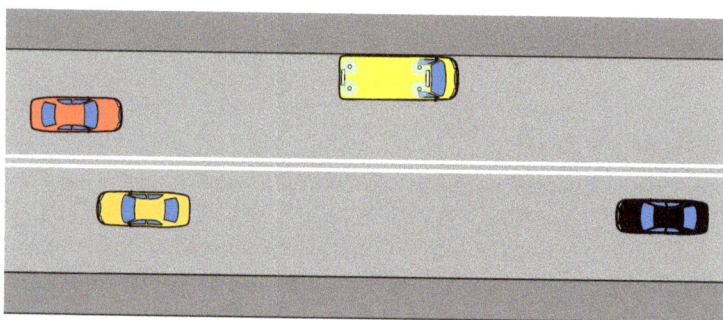

FIGURE 10.2 • Parking within an area controlled by double white lines.

Leaving the Engine Running While the Vehicle is Unattended

Regulation 107(2)(a), **Road Vehicles (Construction and Use) Regulations 1986**

- Always ensure that you have the correct PPE when exiting the vehicle.
- Consider vehicle security – is it fitted with a 'run-lock' facility?
- Could the vehicle's engine overheat?
- Could engine fumes present issues?
- Could engine noise create issues to residents?
- Consider the environmental impact of leaving the engine idling for long periods of time.

Parking on the Offside During the Hours of Darkness
Regulation 101(2)(a), **Road Vehicles (Construction and Use) Regulations 1986**

- Always ensure that you have the correct PPE when exiting the vehicle.
- Leave position (sidelights) illuminated, but turn off vehicle's headlights.
- Consider use of hazard warning lights.
- Leaving a vehicle in a dangerous position is an offence and an exemption to this cannot be claimed.
- Note the danger of using offside vehicle lockers and side door.
- Remember the side step may intrude into path of vehicles.

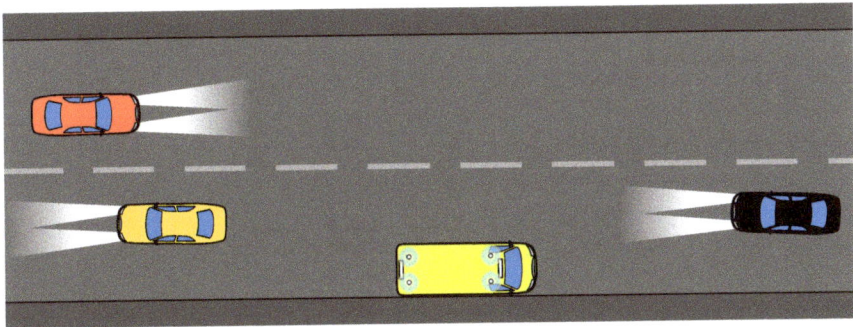

FIGURE 10.3 • Parking on the offside of the road at night.

Parking or Driving on a Cycle Track
Section 21(2)(a), **Road Traffic Act 1988**

- Always ensure that you have the correct PPE when exiting the vehicle.
- Consider possible obstructions to cyclists and pedestrians.
- Be mindful of damage to tyres and suspension, as well the kerb and paving.
- Consider use of hazard warning lights.
- Leaving a vehicle in a dangerous position is an offence and an exemption to this cannot be claimed.
- Be aware that high kerbs may create a large degree of tilt.
- Be aware of potential issues with tail lift or ramp, particularly if the ground is soft.
- Be mindful of the fact that a verge may be unstable or have a slippery surface.

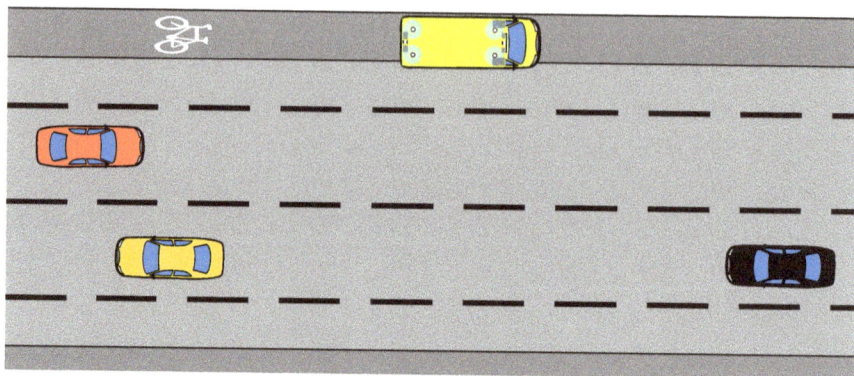

FIGURE 10.4 • Parking or driving on a cycle track.

Parking at a Designated Bus Stop

Schedule 7, Part 6, Paragraph 4(1)(d), **The Traffic Signs Regulations and General Directions 2016**

- Always ensure that you have the correct PPE when exiting the vehicle.
- Consider possible obstructions to pedestrians.
- Consider disruption to buses, particularly if passengers are unable to board or alight.
- Consider use of hazard warning lights.
- Leaving a vehicle in a dangerous position is an offence and an exemption to this cannot be claimed.

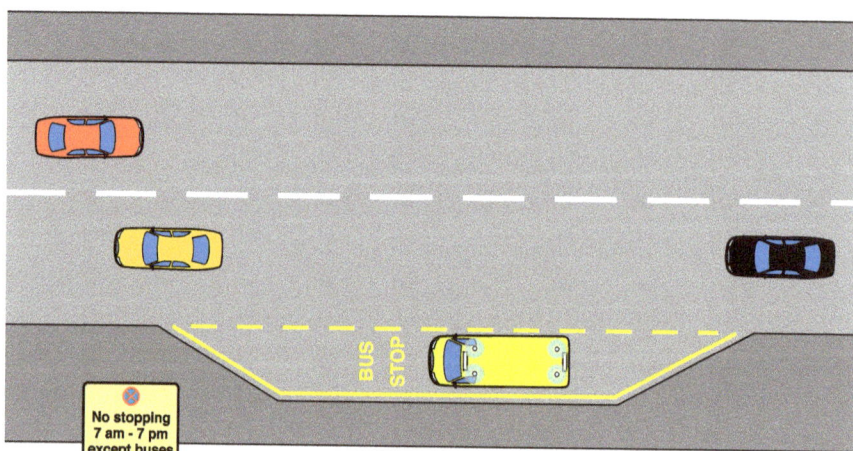

FIGURE 10.5 • Parking at a designated bus stop.

Double Parking or Parking Across a Dropped Kerb

Double parking: *Section 85(3),* **Traffic Management Act 2004**

Parking across a dropped kerb: *Section 86(4),* **Traffic Management Act 2004**

- Always ensure that you have the correct PPE when exiting the vehicle.
- Consider possible obstructions to traffic trying to pass, especially larger vehicles.
- Consider possible obstruction to traffic trying to enter/exit premises.
- Consider seeking the permission of the driveway owner, if parking across a dropped kerb.
- Could an ambulance or fire engine pass?
- Consider use of hazard warning lights.
- Leaving a vehicle in a dangerous position is an offence and an exemption to this cannot be claimed.
- Consider leaving a contact number on the windscreen if possible.

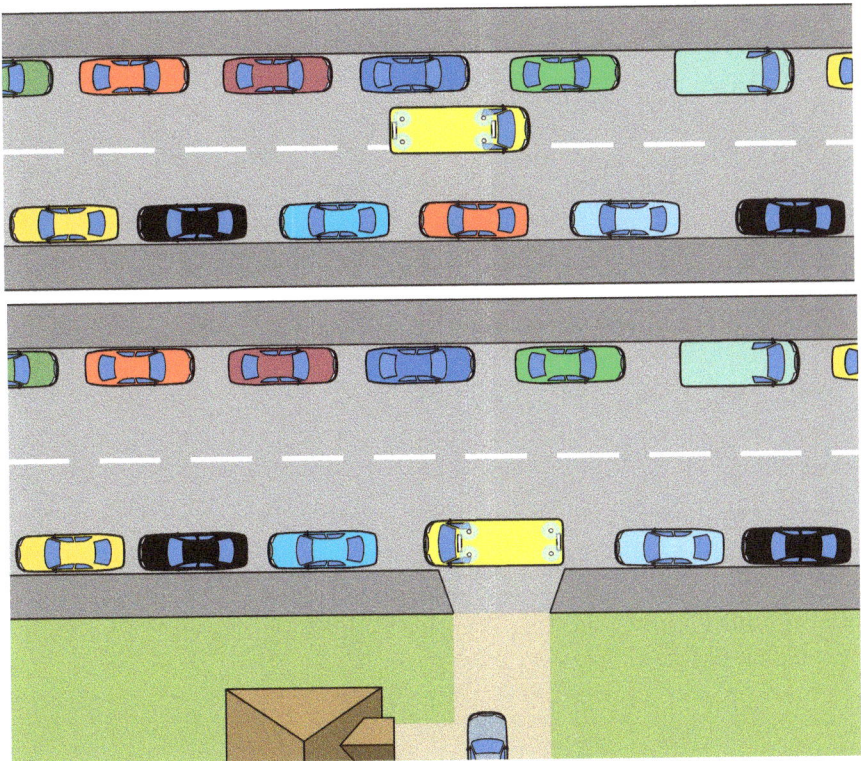

FIGURE 10.6 • Double parking or parking on a dropped kerb.

Parking Within Yellow Zig-zag Markings at Schools, Entrances etc.

- Always ensure that you have the correct PPE when exiting the vehicle.
- Consider possible obstructions to pedestrians (particularly parents and children at schools).
- Consider possible obstruction to traffic trying to enter/exit premises.
- Consider seeking the permission of the property owner, if parking across an entrance.
- It is an offence to leave a vehicle in a dangerous position, for which there is no exemption.

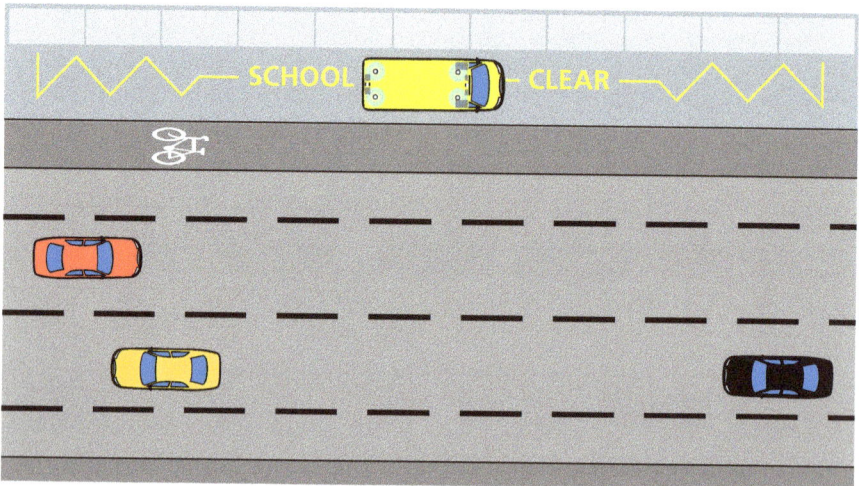

FIGURE 10.7 • Parking Within Yellow Zig-zag Markings at School, Entrances etc.

Exemptions While Engaged on an Emergency Response

Travelling on the Incorrect Side of a 'Keep Left' or 'Keep Right' Sign

Schedule 3, Part 4, Paragraph 3(c), **The Traffic Signs Regulations and General Directions 2016**

- These signs are normally accompanied by bollards and central refuges.
- Be aware of pedestrians using these areas.
- Ensure opposing vehicles have responded before passing on the incorrect side of the signs.
- Speed should be reduced.
- Pedestrians may be looking the wrong way for your direction of travel.

- Be aware of the dangers of returning to the correct road positioning – use of mirrors and signals is essential.

Exceeding Statutory Speed Limits

Section 87(1)(1), **Road Traffic Regulation Act 1984**

- Danger of 'red mist' affecting the driver.
- Speed should be related to available space and presence of hazards.
- You must be able to stop on your own side of the road within the distance that can be seen to be clear.
- You must comply with the organisation's policy in relation to exceeding speed limits.
- Speed of approach must give other road users time to react.
- Speed must be appropriate to the prevailing road and weather conditions.
- You must be aware of your own and the vehicle's limitations.

Red mist

The term is used to describe a psychological state that can arise when drivers of emergency response vehicles are travelling at speed, focusing on what may be presented at the incident they are travelling to, rather than their driving. It can cloud one's ability to assess driving risks realistically and to make the logical decisions essential for the safety of the crew and other road users.

Treating a Red Traffic Light as a 'Give Way', Including Light Controlled Crossing and Temporary Lights

Schedule 14, Part 1, Paragraph 5(6)(c), **The Traffic Signs Regulations and General Directions 2016**

- Your actions must not cause other road users to pass through a red traffic signal.
- The speed of approach must provide other road users with the time to see hear and react to the responding vehicle.
- Are all other road users aware of the presence of the emergency vehicle?
- If there is no path for the response vehicle to pass through the red light, you must stop short of the junction by approximately eight car lengths and consider turning off audible and visual warning equipment to prevent any vehicles in front from entering the junction. Leaving a gap of approximately eight car lengths ensures you are still visible to other traffic. This method, sometimes referred to as 'effective non-use', helps maintain control of the scene and avoids encouraging unsafe movements from other road users. It ensures both public and response vehicle safety whilst allowing the ability to respond promptly once conditions allow.
- You should not go beyond the stop line in a manner, or at a time, likely to endanger anyone.

- You should not cause the driver of any vehicle proceeding in accordance with the indications of light signals to change its speed or course in order to avoid an accident.
- Consider that other emergency vehicles may be entering the junction on a green traffic signal.
- At pedestrian controlled lights, always give precedence to any pedestrian showing an intention to cross.
- Use early vehicle positioning to indicate your intended route.
- Use all warning equipment.
- Keep scanning left and right as you cross through the junction.

Use of Audible Warning Instruments at Night on a Restricted Road Between 23:30–07:00 Hours

Regulation 99(1)(5) and 37(5), **Road Vehicles (Construction and Use) Regulations 1986**

- Consider use of other audible devices
- Use must be relative to the presence of other road users
- Where audible warning equipment is not being used, reduce speed near hazards
- Non-use of audible warning equipment must be justifable (see Chapter 11 on **Audible and Visual Warnings**).

Stopping Within a Yellow Box Junction

Schedule 9, Part 7, Paragraph 11(5)(c), **The Traffic Signs Regulations and General Directions 2016**

Stopping on a yellow box junction may prevent other vehicles from clearing the junction.

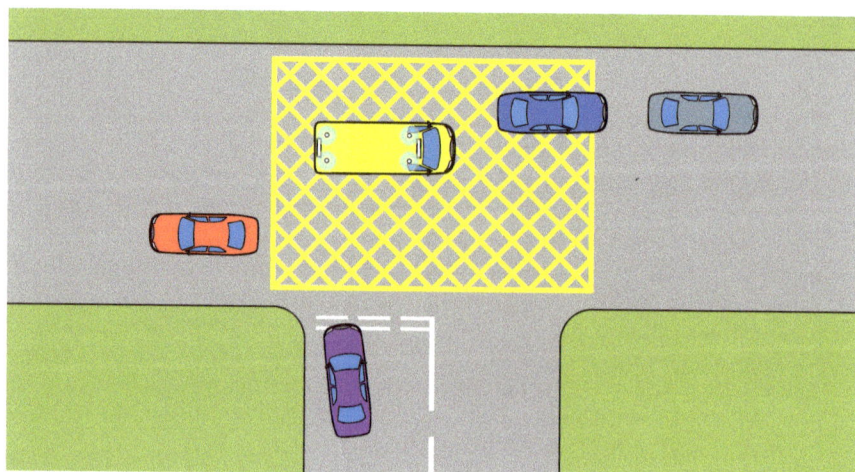

FIGURE 10.8 • Stop within the confines of a yellow box junction.

Driving in Mandatory With-flow Cycle Lanes

- Be aware of pedal cycles using the cycle lane.
- Consider other road users may move left into a cycle lane in response to an emergency response vehicle.

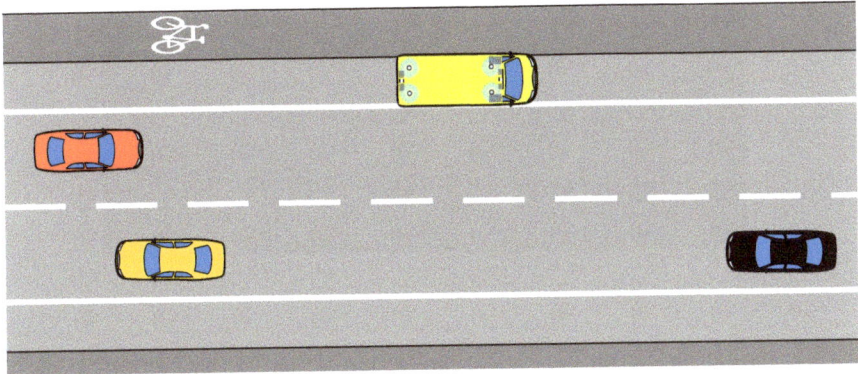

Motorway Regulations

Section 16(1)(d), **Motorway Traffic (England and Wales) Regulations 1982**

The following exemptions can be claimed in order to avoid or prevent an accident, or to obtain or give help required at an accident scene:

- Direction of driving
- Drive on the carriageway only
- Restriction of stopping
- Restriction on reversing
- Restriction of use of hard shoulder
- Restriction on use of central reservation or verge.

There are several ways in which motorway driving differs to that of other roads.

- Be aware of higher speeds involved.
- Sirens are unlikely to be as effective.
- There are fast road policies to be complied with.
- Use of PPE is essential.
- Be aware of higher vulnerability, especially when stationary.
- Understand how new 'smart' motorways work.

Motorway signs

Schedule 15, Part I, Paragraph 5(a), **Traffic Signs Regulations and General Directions 2016**

Do not proceed any further in this lane

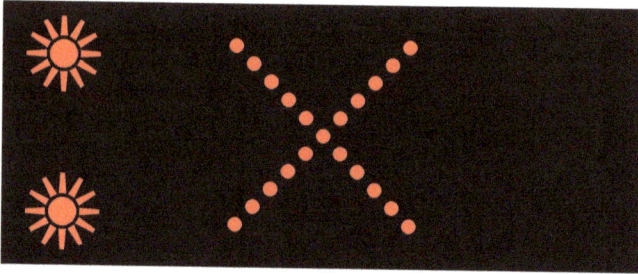

FIGURE 10.10 • Motorway sign: Do not proceed any further in this lane.

Leave motorway at next exit

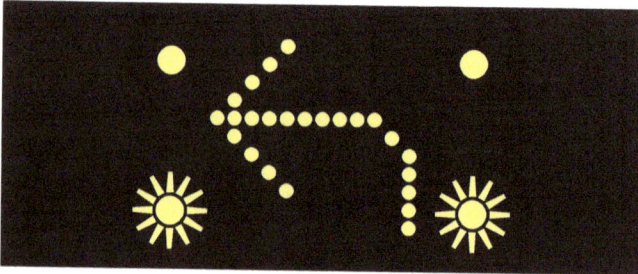

FIGURE 10.11 • Motorway sign: Leave motorway at next exit.

- Be alert as to the location of the actual incident
- Be aware of other emergency vehicles attending the same incident
- Other vehicles may be driving/reversing in the opposite direction to avoid the congestion ahead.

Traffic Regulation Orders

In addition to exemptions written into primary legislation, local authorities can use a Traffic Regulation Order (TRO) to place temporary, experimental or permanent restrictions on traffic within their areas. Though exemptions do exist for the majority of situations in most areas, their application will ultimately be at the discretion of the local authority in which the TRO is situated. The finer details of the provisions applicable to the TRO would have been discussed with the affected services during the consultation period, when the particular TRO was processed and created, and before it formally came into force.

Importantly, without an exemption, it is a criminal offence to contravene a TRO under section 5 of the **Road Traffic Regulation Act 1984**. The legal basis for exemptions derive from section 87 of the same Act and allows emergency vehicles to disregard certain traffic signs and TROs when responding to emergencies where:

- The vehicle is being used for fire brigade, ambulance or police purposes;
- The driver is acting in the course of duty; and
- The disregard is necessary for emergency response.

Routine travel (such as commuting or administrative use) is not exempt and drivers must still exercise due care and caution: the exemption does not absolve liability for reckless driving. It is not possible to predict in every circumstance whether the exemption will apply: if an incident occurs during a breach of a TRO, liability may be assessed based on necessity and proportionality – i.e. the precise circumstances of each case.

Some of the common environments relevant to the driving activities of the ambulance service that are subject to TROs relate to:

Stopping on a Clearway

- Always ensure that you have the correct personal protective equipment (PPE) when exiting the vehicle.
- Consider use of hazard warning lights.
- Leaving a vehicle in a dangerous position is an offence and an exemption to this cannot be claimed.

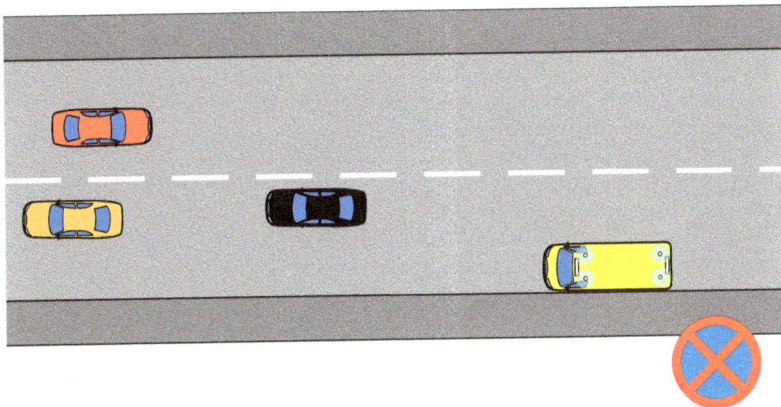

FIGURE 10.12 • Stopping on a clearway.

Parking on a Central Reservation

- Always ensure that you have the correct PPE when exiting the vehicle.
- Consider possible obstructions to pedestrians.
- Consider the close proximity of high-speed traffic.
- There could be possible damage to the vehicle's tyres or suspension.
- Consider whether the ground could be soft, causing potential issues with tail lift/ramp.
- Consider use of hazard warning lights.
- Leaving a vehicle in a dangerous position is an offence and an exemption to this cannot be claimed.
- Be aware that high verges may create a large degree of tilt.
- Be aware that the central reservation may be unstable or have a slippery surface.
- Note the danger of using offside vehicle lockers and side door.
- Remember the side step may intrude into path of vehicles.
- Central crash barriers to prevent cross-over collisions may restrict opening of the driver's door.

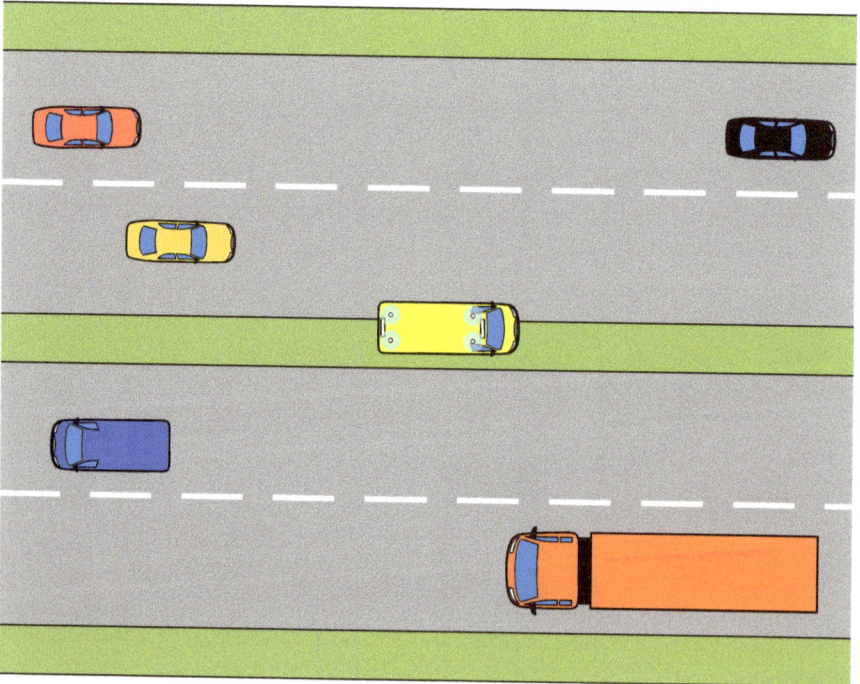

FIGURE 10.13 • Parking on a central reservation.

Bus Lanes

- Be aware of other vehicles using the bus lane.

- Be aware of parked vehicles within the bus lane.

- Consider other road users may move left into a bus lane in response to an emergency response vehicle.

- Consider the bus lane may become obstructed, or end at any time.

Tram Routes

- Always give precedence to trams.

- Consider your use of speed, as the road surface is usually uneven, and rails are slippery when wet.

- Ensure you are familiar with tram light signals. Though they do not apply to vehicles, there is a benefit to understand the light signals, and any possible risk that may be associated with their application.

Parking within Areas Controlled by Double Red or Yellow Lines

- Always ensure you are wearing the correct PPE when exiting the vehicle.

- Consider danger when boarding a patient on a stretcher.

- Keep time parked to a minimum.

- Consider use of hazard warning lights.

- It is an offence to leave a vehicle in a dangerous position, for which there is no exemption.

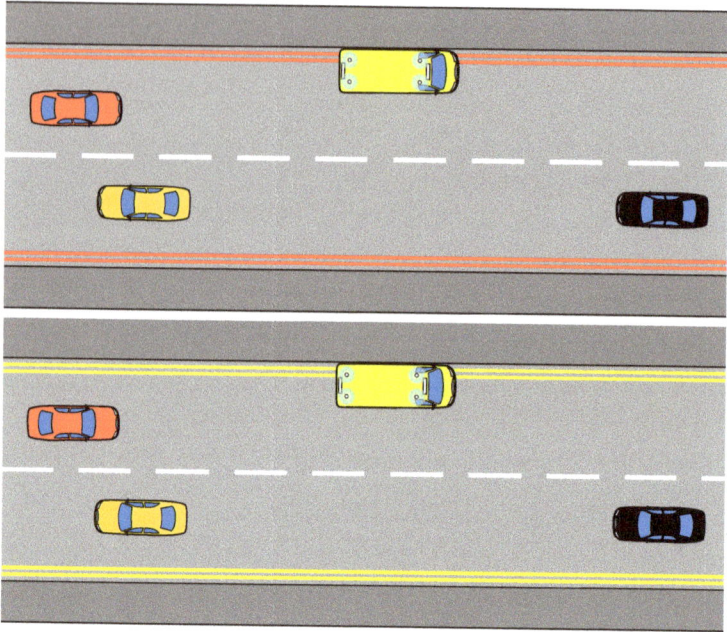

FIGURE 10.14 • Parking within an area controlled by double red lines or double yellow lines.

Pedestrian Precincts

- Extreme caution and slow speed is required due to the proximity of pedestrians.
- You must conform to recognised traffic flow.
- Give pedestrians precedence.
- Be aware of delivery vehicles and their drivers.
- Remember vehicle security is easily compromised in busy areas.
- You should always use a banksman during any reversing manoeuvre, due to the proximity of pedestrians.
- Sirens may be unsuitable due to close proximity of pedestrians.

Low Emission Zones

A Low Emission Zone (LEZ) is a defined area where access by some polluting vehicles is restricted or deterred with the aim of improving air quality. In cities like London, the LEZ encourages drivers and vehicle operators to become cleaner by imposing charges for vehicles which do not meet emission standards throughout the area at all times. The following points should be considered with regards to LEZs.

- **Emission zones relating to ambulance vehicles:**

  When ambulance drivers enter an LEZ, they should follow specific guidelines to minimize emissions and comply with environmental regulations

- **Understand the LEZ rules:**

  Familiarize yourself with the LEZ boundaries, operating hours, and emissions standards. Different cities or regions may have varying criteria for LEZs.

- **Vehicle compliance:**

  Fleet managers should ensure ambulances meet the LEZ emissions standards. If it doesn't meet the LEZ standards, they should consider upgrading to a compliant vehicle.

- **Plan routes:**

  For non-emergency response, consider route planning tools to avoid LEZs if your ambulance doesn't meet the emission requirements. Identify alternative routes to minimize time spent within the zone.

- **Fuel-efficient driving:**

  Encourage drivers to adopt fuel-efficient habits: smooth acceleration, reduced idling, and maintaining optimal tyre pressure. These practices reduce emissions.

- **Zero-emission vehicles:**

  If available, use zero-emission ambulances (electric) within the LEZ. Many ambulance services are transitioning to such vehicles.

- **Regular maintenance:**

  Keep your ambulance well-maintained. Regular servicing ensures optimal engine performance and minimises emissions.

Remember, LEZs aim to improve air quality and public health, so following these guidelines benefits both the environment and patients. Most Ambulance Service/Trust have local agreements to ensure that all ambulance vehicles are exempt from charges within the LEZ. Check with ambulance control, fleet department, or your local policy, to ensure your vehicle is not charged whilst entering and negotiating the LEZ, when travelling to or from another service/trust.

Double White Lines Where the Line Nearest You is Solid

There is a misconception, in some quarters, that an exemption exists that permits emergency response drivers to contravene a solid white line system.

The law is very clear: the only exemptions that exist are those that are available to the general public.

These exemptions are detailed in the *Schedule 9, Part 7, Paragraph 5,* **The Traffic Signs Regulations and General Directions 2016**. They are:

- To enable the vehicle to enter, from the side of the road on which it is proceeding, or the land or premises adjacent to the length of road on which the line is placed, or another road joining that road
- In order to pass a stationary vehicle
- Owing to circumstances outside the control of the driver
- In order to avoid an accident
- In order to pass a road maintenance vehicle that is in use, is moving at a speed not exceeding 10 mph and is displaying to the rear a 'keep right' sign
- In order to pass a pedal cycle moving at a speed not exceeding 10 mph
- In order to pass a horse that is being ridden or led at a speed not exceeding 10 mph
- For the purposes of complying with any direction of a constable in uniform or a traffic warden.

Other than in any of the circumstances outlined above, if a driver was to cross or straddle a double white line, where the solid white line is nearest to them, they would be guilty of an offence.

Legal Exemptions in Summary

Exemptions Which Apply for any Category of Patient

- Parking within the controlled (zig-zag) area of a pedestrian crossing
- Parking within areas controlled be double white lines
- Leaving the engine running while the vehicle is unattended
- Parking on the offside during the hours of darkness
- Parking or driving on a cycle track
- Parking at a designated bus stop
- Double parking
- Parking across a dropped kerb
- Parking within yellow zig-zag markings at school, entrances etc.

Exemptions Which Apply Whilst Engaged on an Emergency Response

- Travelling on the incorrect side of a 'keep left' or 'keep right' sign
- Exceeding statutory speed limits
- Treating a red traffic light as a 'give way', including light controlled crossing and temporary lights
- Use of audible warning instruments at night
- Stopping within a yellow box junction
- Driving in mandatory with-flow cycle lanes
- Motorway regulations

Traffic Regulation Orders (TROs)

- Stopping on a clearway
- Parking on a central reservation
- Bus lanes
- Tram routes
- Parking within areas controlled by double red or yellow lines
- Pedestrian precincts
- Low emission zones

(?) **KNOWLEDGE RECAP**

1 List the exemptions that are available to an ambulance driver when responding to emergencies.
2 What questions should a driver ask themselves prior to exercising any exemption?
3 Is there any exemption that allows a response driver to park in a dangerous position?
4 Is there a specific exemption for an emergency response driver to cross or straddle a solid white nearest to them on a double white line system?

CHAPTER 11

Audible and Visual Warnings

LEARNING OUTCOMES

By the end of this chapter you should:

- Understand the purpose and use of passive visual warnings.
- Understand the purpose and use of active visual warnings.
- Understand the purpose and use of audible warnings.
- Recognise the benefit of alternating siren tones.
- Recognise when the use of emergency warning equipment (EWE) is permitted.
- Recognise when EWE must not be used and when the deactivation of sirens should be considered.

The presence of an emergency vehicle often influences the behaviour of other road users and pedestrians and, for these reasons, emergency ambulances are fitted with visual or audible warnings, or both, to alert road users to your presence or approach.

In this chapter we consider the active and passive visual warnings that are incorporated into ambulances, as well as their audible warnings, and the impact that they can have on other road users.

Appearance and Markings

There are two types of visual warning on an ambulance. These are passive or active.

Passive Visual Warnings

Modern emergency vehicles are fitted with retro-reflective high contrast colour passive visual warnings, which reflect light from car headlights. Emergency ambulances are usually painted yellow to meet the requirements of the CEN 1789:2007 European Union Standard for ambulances and medical transportation vehicles (the UK equivalent is BS EN 1789:2007).

The word 'ambulance' is depicted in mirror image format on the front of the vehicle using the retro-reflective material to enable drivers in front of the approaching ambulance to identify it in their mirrors.

Emergency vehicles are equipped with 'checkerboard' or 'Battenberg' markings along the length of the vehicle. The colours yellow and green are reserved for use by the ambulance service only. Similarly the police may use blue and yellow, the fire and rescue service uses red and yellow and National Highways uses black and yellow. Note that in other parts of the UK the police or other agencies may take on the role of National Highways. In order for any retro-reflective material to remain effective it is important that the vehicle is kept clean.

Further information regarding the correct use of retro-reflective markings can be found in the **Road Vehicles Lighting Regulations 1989**, schedules 17 and 18.

It is important to remember that the bright yellow colouring and markings on ambulances may suddenly be noticed by traffic ahead of you. This can sometimes be after a prolonged period of non-observance, resulting in sudden or unexpected vehicle movement or braking without warning. It is therefore important that adequate following distances are maintained.

Active Visual Warnings

These warning lights commonly include flashing blue lights – white and blue strobes and LEDs fitted to the roof, front, sides and rear. Flashing headlights can be used during daylight hours. The emergency warning lights must have 360° visibility around the vehicle in order to be BS EN 1789 compliant.

Blue flashing lights are only permitted to be used by services specifically defined in the **Road Vehicles Lighting Regulations 1989**, as amended by the **Deregulation Act 2015**.

For flashing headlights, the majority of modern emergency vehicles have the facility to disable, or have an inbuilt feature that prevents, this type of warning light from being activated at night when the vehicle headlights are switched on. This minimises the risk of dazzling other drivers.

Some ambulance services that serve the UK's airports may have airport beacons fitted to their emergency vehicles. These are yellow or amber in colour and should only be used when the vehicle is deployed at the airport's 'airside'.

Audible Warnings

Sirens

Most modern ambulances are fitted with electronic sirens that have the benefit of alerting people to the presence of an ambulance before they are able to see it. Sirens can usually produce a range of different noises/tones that can be useful in different situations, for example:

- **'Wail' sound:** characterised by a long up and down variation with an unbroken tone, the 'wail' siren is best used when traveling on a long stretch of road or in open areas. The long slow tone is spread out from the front of the vehicle in a fan shape.
- **'Yelp' sound:** this is similar to the 'wail' siren but faster, emitting the familiar 'whoo-whoo-whoo-whoo' sound. The 'yelp' siren is preferred in heavy slow traffic, at junctions and in built up areas. The fast short tones of the yelp siren bounce off buildings, cars and other structures to deflect the noise, but this can cause confusion among other road users as to the direction of approach of the emergency vehicle.
- **'Pulsar' (Phaser/Piercer) sound:** delivering a rapid, high-pitched tone designed to cut through ambient noise in high-traffic situations or built-up areas. Its sharp, oscillating pitch helps the vehicle stand out, ensuring maximum attention and effectiveness in both directional and 360-degree sound applications. This alerts road users from all angles, enabling them to pinpoint the direction of the approaching ambulance.

There might possibly be a fourth tone, such as **'french horn'**. Ambulance services may specifically train their drivers to use different siren tones in different situations, so refer to your local policy. A **'bull horn'** if fitted provides a completely different non-electronic baritone warning. This is often used to supplement the 'normal' emergency audible warning sounds. These can be useful to attract attention but should never be used in an aggressive manner.

Emergency Warning Equipment in Practice

Drivers of emergency vehicles have a duty to warn other road users of their presence and intentions by exposing, to those who would benefit, any warning equipment – visual or audible – that is fitted to the vehicle. This should be balanced against the occasions when it offers more protection to deactivate audible and visual warning equipment, for example when in standing traffic where it can be intimidating.

Blue flashing lights and sirens influence the behaviour of other road users – this is due to the presence of the emergency vehicle and the urgency of the journey being undertaken. They do not give any legal entitlement to claim precedence where it is unsafe. You should also be aware at all times that if you have EWE fitted to a vehicle, the public have the right to receive the warning the equipment is designed to give.

The nature of loud sirens may be intimidating, so they must be used intelligently in stationary traffic when there is a risk of threatening or forcing other vehicles to commit to a potentially dangerous manoeuvre that they may not have attempted otherwise. In this case, deactivation of the EWE must be considered (effective non-use).

In the event of a response driver remaining with the patient en route to the hospital (due to their advanced clinical skills, for example), one of the ambulance crew members may be asked to drive the response vehicle to the receiving hospital. When this situation arises, the response vehicle must not utilise EWE and must adhere to all road traffic regulations. The response vehicle must not act as an escort to the ambulance.

If you believe that the vehicle in front may not have heard the siren, changing the siren tone may gain their attention. However, you should refrain from repeatedly flicking between the siren tones as this may be perceived as aggressive or intimidating to the other road user.

---

⑦ KNOWLEDGE RECAP

1 Describe an emergency vehicle's passive visual warnings.
2 Describe an emergency vehicle's active visual warnings.
3 Different siren tones can be beneficial in different situations. When might it be preferable to use a 'yelp' setting rather than a 'wail' setting?
4 In what circumstances should the deactivation of sirens be considered and why?

CHAPTER 12

Lighting Regulations

LEARNING OUTCOMES

By the end of this chapter you should:

- Know the exceptional circumstances under which it is legal to have lights that are not in full working order.
- Know which vehicles may be fitted with a blue flashing light.
- Know when it is legally acceptable to use your blue flashing lights.
- Understand the amendments made to the **Road Vehicles Lighting Regulations** in 2005.
- Understand the amendments made to the **Road Vehicles Lighting and Goods Vehicle (Plating and Testing) (amendment) Regulations 2009**.
- Be able to access full versions of the **Road Vehicles Lighting Regulations**.

The Road Vehicles Lighting Regulations 1989 (and amendments made in 2005) and the **Road Vehicles Lighting and Goods Vehicle (Plating and Testing) (amendment) Regulations 2009** detail the requirements for how and when motor vehicles should be lit on public roads. Drivers of emergency response vehicles must be aware of these rules and, in particular, the specific regulations associated to the use and restrictions of emergency warning lights and retro-reflective markings.

This chapter provides a summary of these regulations and their amendments, and links to the full legislation for further reading.

Road Vehicles Lighting Regulations 1989

The information provided in this chapter briefly outlines the regulations for general lighting and the use of emergency warning lighting and retro-reflective materials, on emergency vehicles.

Drivers should remember that legislation is periodically updated and that it is their responsibility to keep up to date with any changes.

General Rules

All lights, lamps and reflectors must be clean and in full working order. The only exceptions to this are when:

- The light, lamp or reflector has stopped working on your current journey.
- Arrangements have been made to remedy the defect.
- You are towing a trailer with working lights (so your vehicle's broken light/lamp/reflector cannot be seen).

Blue Warning Beacons

The Road Vehicles Lighting Regulations 1989 (Section 16) state: 'No vehicle, other than an emergency vehicle or a vehicle used for special forces purposes, shall be fitted with:
(a) a blue warning beacon or special warning lamp, or
(b) a device which resembles a blue warning beacon or a special warning lamp, whether the same is in working order or not.'

In line with the **Road Vehicles Lighting Regulations 1989** (Section 27), as the driver of an emergency vehicle you must be able to justify the use of emergency warning equipment; you may use blue flashing lights when:

- You are responding to an incident
- You are at the scene of an incident to warn of your presence

- To warn others of your approach or presence on the road
- To let people know that there is a hazard on the road
- To facilitate the medical treatment of a patient with urgent need.

Changes Made in 2005

In 2005, a number of changes were made to the lighting regulations. They can be summarised as follows:

1 Emergency vehicles are no longer defined as having to have a motor, thereby permitting non-motor emergency vehicles to use blue flashing lights, for example bicycles and electric vehicles.

2 Flashing lights may be used on bicycles (one to four flashes per second, with an equal amount of time on and off, in the usual colours of white to the front and red to the rear). The exemption for the use of blue flashing lights for a bicycle is now extended.

Retro-Reflective Material

The regulations pertaining to the correct and proper use of retro-reflective material are contained within Part 2 of Schedule 17 and 18 of the **Road Vehicles Lighting Regulations 1989**, the 2009 regulations and the **Deregulation Act 2015**.

Statutory ambulance service vehicles are permitted to use red, yellow or orange reflectors to the rear. In the case of vehicles owned by a statutory ambulance service, or held on a lease or hire agreement by them, the side reflectors may be amber, yellow, green or white, or if within 1 metre of the rear of the vehicle they may be red.

Fire, police and traffic officers are also allocated protected colours for side retro-reflective materials under the 2009 regulations.

Finding Road Vehicles Lighting Regulations Online

The links provided below give additional information on lighting regulations relating to ambulance vehicles. Legislation changes frequently so you should ensure that you use the most up-to-date information that can be found on the government legislation website.

Road Vehicles Lighting Regulations 1989
www.legislation.gov.uk/uksi/1989/1796/made

Road Vehicles Lighting (Amendment) Regulations 2005
www.legislation.gov.uk/uksi/2005/2559/contents/made

Road Vehicles Lighting (Amendment) (No. 2) Regulations 2005
www.legislation.gov.uk/uksi/2005/3169/contents/made

The Road Vehicles Lighting and Goods Vehicle (Plating and Testing) (amendment) Regulations 2009
www.legislation.gov.uk/uksi/2009/3220/regulation/13/made

Deregulation Act 2015
www.legislation.gov.uk/ukpga/2015/20/schedule/9/enacted

(?) **KNOWLEDGE RECAP**

1 In what circumstances is it acceptable to have lights on a vehicle that are not in full working order?
2 Which vehicles may be fitted with blue flashing lights?
3 Name three situations in which the use of blue flashing lights is permitted.
4 What colour retro-reflective material is an ambulance permitted to use to the front and rear of the vehicle and what conditions are attached to this?

CHAPTER 13

Re-Prioritisation of Calls

LEARNING OUTCOMES

By the end of this chapter you should:

- Be aware of all options available to a driver to turn a vehicle around safely.
- Be able to identify the most appropriate manoeuvre to turn the vehicle around safely in any given situation.
- Understand the advantages and disadvantages with each of the options.

There will be occasions when a driver will need to turn their vehicle around promptly. An example would be in the event of receiving a higher category emergency call requiring the vehicle to return along the route that it has just travelled. The manoeuvre must be conducted safely, without risk of damage to any road user or property. In the absence of a nearby roundabout, the most efficient way to turn a vehicle around is to conduct a 'U' turn.

The ability to complete this manoeuvre will depend on the size of the vehicle, the steering lock available, street furniture, width of road and the actual or potential presence of other vehicles (moving or stationary).

Drivers can consider the use of emergency warning equipment to complete any of these manoeuvres, provided the reason for the turn justifies its use.

'U' Turn

A driver can consider using a 'U' turn where the road width and the absence of other dangers allow this tactic. It may be necessary for the driver to pull over to the nearside to allow other vehicles present to pass before completing the exercise. Emergency equipment should be utilised after the turn is completed to reduce confusion.

The advantage of this tactic is that the manoeuvre can be completed without entering other roads, reversing or causing other motorists to change course or speed.

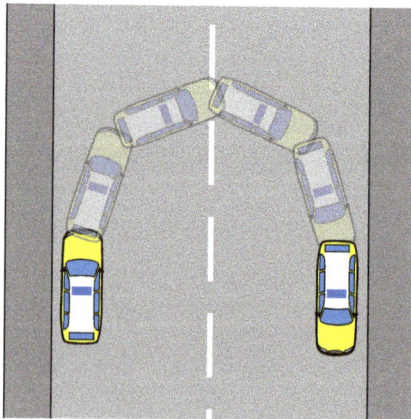

FIGURE 13.1 • A 'U' turn.

Junction 'U' Turns

A driver can consider the use of either a nearside or offside junction to complete a 'U' turn. Prior to and throughout such an action, the driver must ensure that all vehicles present are not confused by their actions. Other road users should be given time to react. The main advantage of a 'U' turn is that the vehicle at no time needs to be reversed.

The preferred option is the use of a junction on the offside. This is because the driver will only have one line of traffic to concede to when re-entering the major road across the 'give way' or 'stop' line.

Drivers must remember that in both scenarios they are potentially crossing the path of traffic approaching the junction.

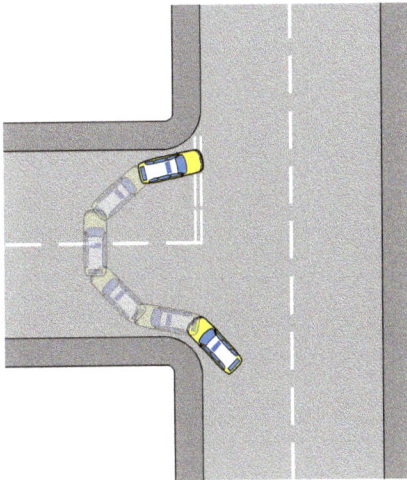

Using a nearside junction

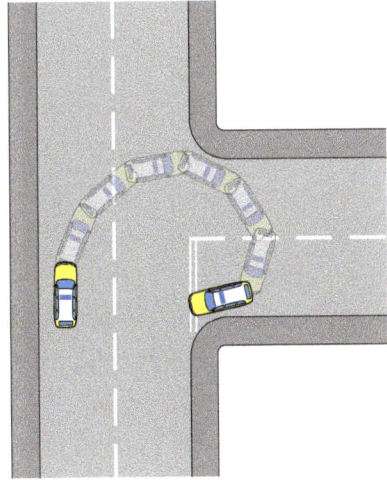

Using an offside junction

FIGURE 13.2 • Junction 'U' turns.

Turn in the Road

A turn in the road should be completed using the minimum number of turns necessary based on the width of the road. It's crucial to observe the surroundings both before and during the manoeuvre.

If the road is wide enough, the turn can be made without stopping on the nearside. However, if the road is narrower, it may be necessary to stop close to and parallel to the nearside verge or kerb to ensure the turn can be safely completed. Always ensure a clear view of oncoming traffic and any potential obstacles throughout the process. This manoeuvre increases the level of risk compared to a U-turn, as it involves reversing within the exercise, which requires additional caution such as effective rearward observations and blind spot checks. Use of a banksman must be considered.

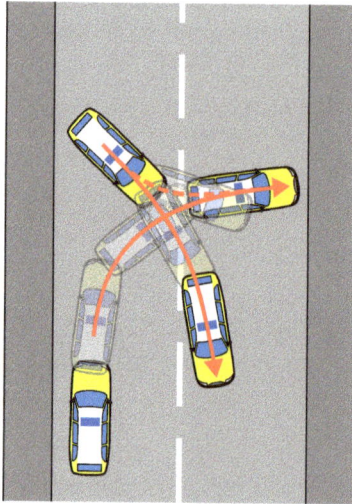

FIGURE 13.3 • Turn in the road.

Junction Reverses

Drivers can consider the use of both nearside and offside minor junctions to reverse their vehicle into the mouth of these junctions. In both cases drivers of emergency vehicles must be sure that all other road users present are not confused by their actions. Drivers must ensure that the speed at which they conduct these manoeuvres allow other road users time to react to their actions.

The preferred option is the offside junction. This is because when the driver reaches the 'give way' or 'stop' line, they will only have one line of traffic to concede to.

Remember that in both scenarios, the emergency vehicle is potentially reversing towards approaching traffic. Use of a banksman must be considered to provide additional warning to other road users.

The 'U' turn option is favourable to the reversing option.

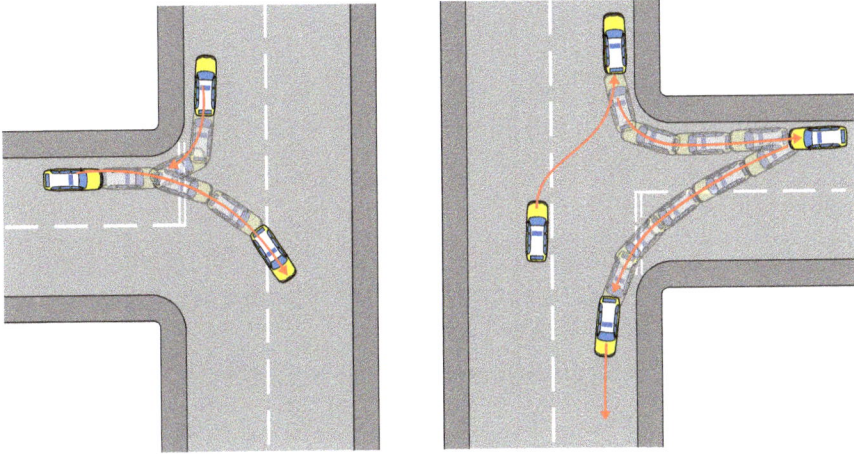

FIGURE 13.4 • Junction reverses.

(?) KNOWLEDGE RECAP

1 What is the advantage of using a 'U' turn over a junction reverse?
2 Why is an offside junction better than a nearside junction for a 'U' turn?
3 When would you consider using a turn in the road?

CHAPTER 14

Attending Incidents

LEARNING OUTCOMES

By the end of this chapter you should:

- Understand the importance of personal protective equipment.
- Understand the importance of scene preservation at serious or fatal road traffic accidents.
- Know how to approach motorway or dual carriageway incidents when traffic is moving slowly or is stationary.
- Know the precautions that must be taken when driving on the hard shoulder.
- Know how to approach motorway or dual carriageway incidents when the carriageway is blocked or closed.
- Understand why travelling in convoy should be avoided and the precautions that must be taken when it is unavoidable.
- Know the safest position in which to park when attending incidents on the motorway or dual carriageway.
- Understand the importance of regular situation reports to ambulance control.
- Know the best practice procedures for leaving a scene.
- Know what to do if you come across an incident when driving a non-emergency vehicle for your trust.
- Know the circumstances in which a police escort may be required and the procedure to follow.

A consistent, uniform approach to attending incidents on multi-lane carriageways (motorways/dual carriageways) and other roads by the emergency services is essential.

Topics covered include strategies to be used when approaching, parking at and leaving incidents on multi-lane carriageways and smaller roads, as well as specific procedures to be followed when you are the first emergency vehicle on scene, travelling in convoy or are accompanied by a police escort.

Dual carriageways may have many of the same characteristics as a motorway, such as hard shoulders, central reservations and speed limits. While their designations are different, the principles applied to motorways should equally be applied to dual carriageways. The term 'fast road' defines any road with a speed limit greater than 40 mph.

Personal Protective Equipment

Personal protective equipment (PPE) – including a fastened high-visibility jacket and hard helmet – should be worn at every incident, no matter how minor it may seem. This is especially true when attending an incident on a multi-lane carriageway motorway/dual carriageway or any other class of road. Serious head injuries can be – and have been – sustained by members of the emergency services who have been struck by objects thrown up by vehicles passing at high speeds.

Staff should decide whether any further protection is required when carrying out their risk assessment of the incident.

Scene preservation

It is important to remember that the scene of any serious or fatal road traffic accident is considered a crime scene by the police. Although it should not interfere with the care and treatment of patients, which is paramount, you should be mindful, when on scene, to minimise unnecessary disturbance to potential evidence.

Multi-Agency Vehicle Response

Most ambulance response drivers won't be specially trained in multi-resource or convoy response driving. However, some drivers who operate in specialist response teams will have received dedicated training on these skills. Where dedicated training has been received the driver will be authorised to operate within that skill set and the training should be followed.

When an ambulance response driver has not received dedicated training in multi-unit response or convoy driving they should refrain from travelling in convoy when engaged in emergency response driving, however it is accepted that on occasions it may not be possible to avoid, for example when responding to a major incident requiring multiple resources.

In the event that a number of emergency vehicles must travel together with untrained convoy response drivers, then extra care and vigilance must be taken by all drivers. Other road users may not be expecting more than one vehicle and may behave unexpectedly to your presence.

If you are the lead response vehicle, undertake the response drive as normal and within your trained skill set. If you are a following response vehicle, you should use a different siren tone to the vehicle ahead of you, and maintain a safe distance from the vehicle ahead. Be especially vigilant for drivers, pedestrians and other road users that might not be expecting another response vehicles. Always be able to stop within the distance you can see to be clear, and do not rely on the road being clear because the response vehicle ahead of you has progressed.

Police-Escorted Convoys

The protocol for the interaction between police-escorted convoys and other emergency blue light vehicles, in particular which vehicles take priority, has been agreed by the chief officer groups and driver training advisory groups of the police, NHS ambulance service, and fire and rescue services.

Police escorts may be given for a number of reasons including:

- Movement of abnormal loads
- Secure movement of protected persons and very high-risk loads
- Control of road events such as demonstrations
- Facilitating an emergency response by other vehicles (e.g. ambulance escorts)

Where the route is not preplanned or has not been shared in advance, it is common for emergency vehicles to encounter temporary traffic holds directed by police officers engaged on such escorts.

In all cases, any emergency vehicle driver who encounters a police-escorted convoy must comply with directions given by the escorting police officers. Section 35, Road Traffic Act 1988 applies as it does to any temporary road closure directed by a constable in uniform; there is no exemption for emergency drivers. Emergency vehicles are required to comply with directions given by the escorting officers until the convoy has passed, typically within a few seconds.

Secure protection escorts will retain priority for security and safety reasons. Emergency drivers should not attempt to enter, cross, join or overtake the convoy. It would not be possible for escorting officers to verify the status of emergency vehicles and rule out 'trojan horse' attacks within the limited reaction time available to them.

For other types of escort, police may facilitate or prioritise the progress of the emergency vehicle if it is safe, proportionate, and practicable to do so. Responding drivers should bear in mind that in many cases it will be quicker to allow a convoy to pass than to bring it to a halt and clear a path through for another emergency vehicle. In other cases, the nature of the vehicles involved and road layout might make it impossible to immediately clear a route past the convoy.

Motorway and Multi-Lane Carriageway Approach

The high volume of vehicles on multi-lane carriageway motorways and dual carriageways, and the speeds at which they travel, present ambulance staff with unique problems. Minor incidents can rapidly expand to involve a large number of vehicles, while any incident may lead to a large build-up of traffic, causing difficulties for approaching emergency response vehicles.

Different methods of approaching incidents on multi-lane carriageways have been devised depending on the traffic conditions.

- **Flowing traffic:** ambulances should approach using the main carriageway whenever possible, usually in lanes two or three (see Figure 14.1). This allows other road users to react in a normal manner, moving left when seeing an approaching ambulance or hearing sirens. Do not use Lane 1 – this could cause drivers to move onto the hard shoulder where other vehicles may have stopped.
- **Traffic on the main carriageway is moving slowly:** approach on the hard shoulder with visual warning equipment activated (blue lights and flashing headlights). The use of sirens has been known to cause drivers to pull onto the hard shoulder, into the path of emergency response vehicles, so consider their use carefully. Remember: you can use your normal road horn to indicate your presence if required.
- **Traffic on the main carriageway is stationary:** approach on the hard shoulder with all EWE activated – blue flashing lights and sirens. However, you must be aware of the danger of members of the public being on the hard shoulder – people sometimes get out of their vehicles to see what's going on or to stretch their legs if they have been in stationary traffic for some time.

Extreme caution is required when driving on the hard shoulder. The surface may have loose grit, oil and other objects present on it that would not normally be found on the main carriageway. Vehicles may be parked on the hard shoulder and, if broken down, may not have lights at night. People walking to or from emergency telephones may also pose a hazard. Your speed must be chosen with due regard for the circumstances.

Follow the instructions of police officers at all times. Traffic officers may also be required to direct traffic (see Appendix 3). The police may direct drivers to turn around and drive back to the previous exit if an incident has led to the complete blockage or closure of the motorway. You will be notified by the police at the junction where vehicles are being directed off the road if this is taking place. The normal rules of the road apply in these circumstances.

Layout of a Multi-Lane Carriageway

The police may also direct you to approach or leave an incident in the wrong direction if the carriageway is blocked or closed. In these circumstances the same procedure applies:

- Drive on the left
- Use visual warning equipment (blue lights and flashing headlights)
- Keep your speed down
- Be aware that other emergency response vehicles may be travelling towards you on the same carriageway.

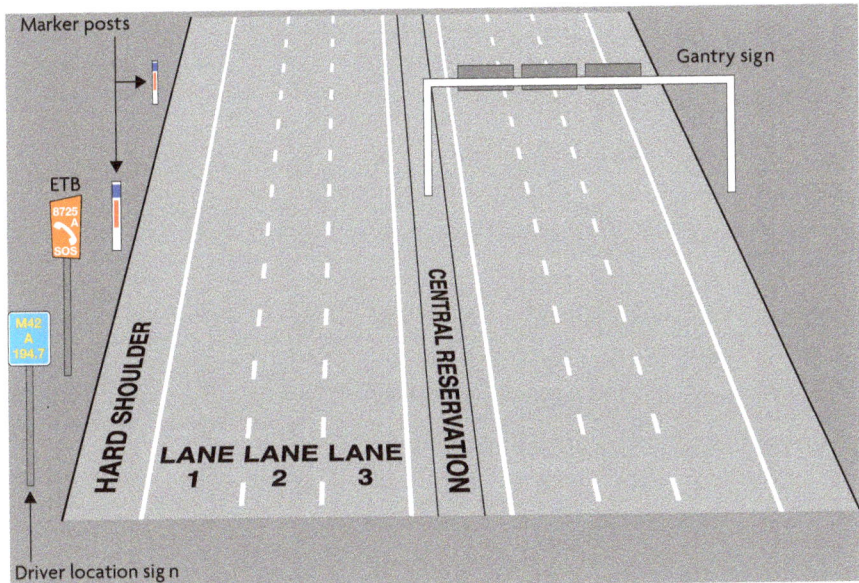

FIGURE 14.1 • Layout of a multi-lane carriageway.

Further guidance on accessing incidents on smart motorways can be found in Chapter 15.

The most commonly used carriageway identifiers are the letters 'A', 'B', 'J', 'K', 'L' and 'M'. Typically the letter 'A' ('Away from London') refers to carriageways heading away from London (or clockwise on the M25 and M60), while the letter 'B' ('Back to London') indicates carriageways heading towards London (anticlockwise on the M25 and M60).

The location matches the one displayed on marker posts. Location numbers increase in the direction of travel of the 'A' carriageway, and decrease along the direction of the 'B' carriageway. The letters 'J', 'K', 'L' and 'M' denote junction slip roads. This is illustrated in Figure 14.2 below.

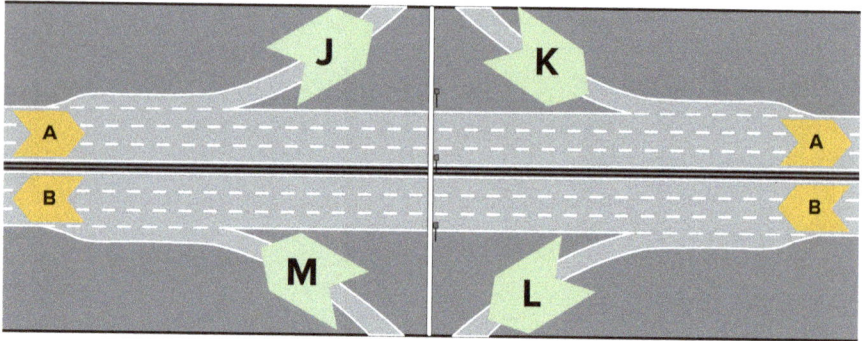

FIGURE 14.2 • Junction slip roads.

Parking on Multi-Lane Carriageways

Crews must perform a risk assessment when arriving on scene, taking the directions of other agencies already present into account to ensure their own safety.

Parking at a Scene Already Protected by the Police or Other Agency

Ambulances will usually be positioned in front of the incident. This will allow the safe loading of casualties for transportation, offer protection from other responding agency vehicles and allow them to leave more quickly. Ultimately, the responsible officer on scene will determine positioning.

Access and egress should be maintained throughout the incident to allow removal of casualties when required. If further vehicles are en route or required, it may be appropriate, following a discussion with the police or National Highways, to position these in front of the incident site in an area that does not obstruct flowing traffic, operations and scene access and egress.

Blue lights and flashing headlights should be turned off when parked within the safe area – doing so significantly reduces the risks arising from 'rubbernecking' motorists. Police or Highways vehicles, which should be parked at the rear of the scene, will provide rear-facing warning lights.

Local procedures

Some local police authorities advocate that emergency vehicles attending motorway or dual carriageway incidents leave all their visual warnings activated. Drivers should be guided by their local organisation's policy.

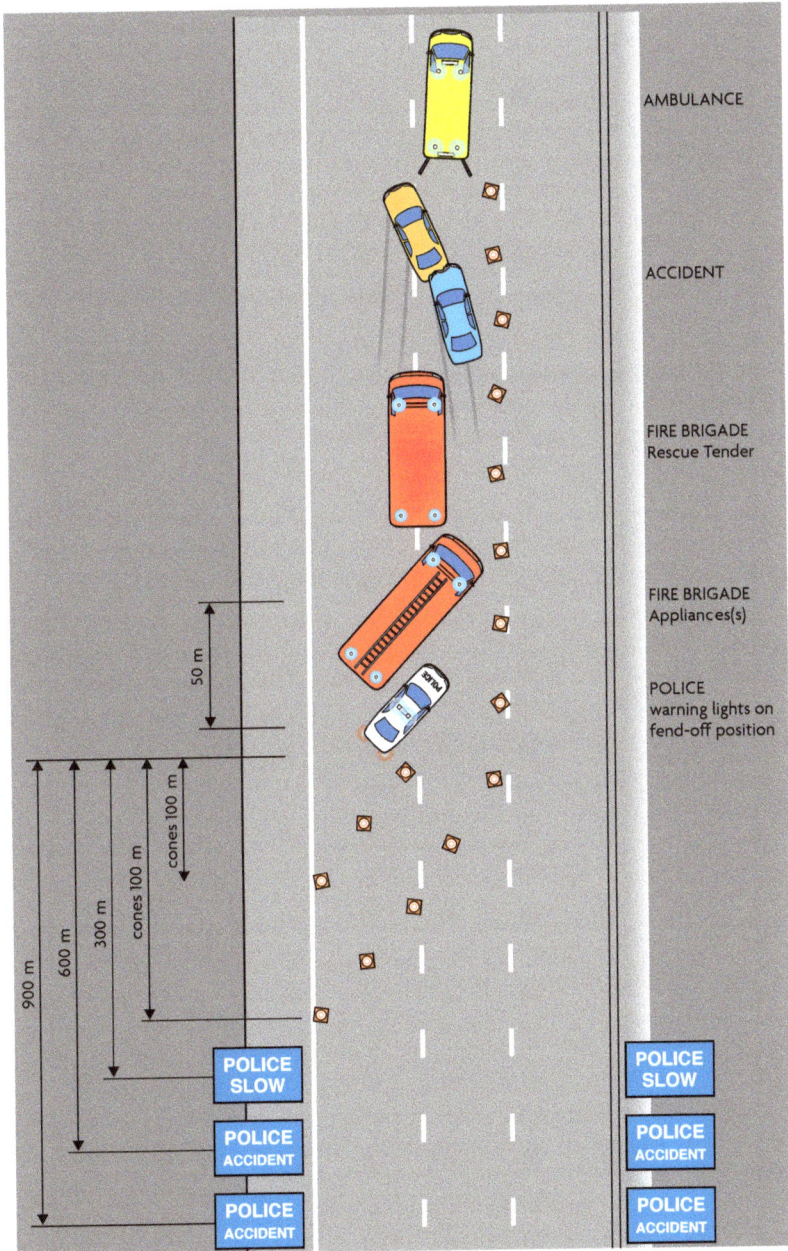

AMBULANCE

ACCIDENT

FIRE BRIGADE
Rescue Tender

FIRE BRIGADE
Appliances(s)

POLICE
warning lights on
fend-off position

50 m

cones 100 m

cones 100 m

300 m

600 m

900 m

POLICE
SLOW

POLICE
ACCIDENT

POLICE
ACCIDENT

POLICE
SLOW

POLICE
ACCIDENT

POLICE
ACCIDENT

FIGURE 14.3 • Parking in a coned-off area.

Ambulance as First Emergency Vehicle on Scene

General guidelines

In all cases stop 50 metres (approximately 12.5 car-lengths) before the incident, turning the front wheels in a safe direction to reduce the risk of the vehicle being pushed into the incident if it is struck. You should also stop in a position that affords maximum visibility of rear visual devices and reflective or high-visibility markings; all rear-facing visual warnings – blue lights, rear-flashing red lights, sidelights, fog lights and hazard lights – should be activated.

Position as detailed below, depending upon which lane the incident is in:

- **Lane 1:** position in Lane 1, do not intrude into Lane 2
- **Lane 2 (three or more lanes):** position in Lanes 1 and 2, normally at an angle (fend-off/in); do not intrude into Lane 3
- **Lane 3:** position in Lane 3 but do not intrude into Lane 2
- **Lanes 2 and 3:** position in Lane 2 and 3; do not intrude into Lane 1.

The police will permit you to block as many lanes as required to ensure your own safety and that of your patients. No one should return to the ambulance once it is parked in a fend-off position unless absolutely necessary.

Keep your eye on passing traffic; you must never assume it is safe. Research has shown that a significant proportion of drivers are unable to distinguish a stationary vehicle from a moving one on a motorway or dual carriageway.

See Appendix 1 for details on Patient Transport and unmarked vehicles attending incidents on motorways and dual carriageways.

Incidents confined to the hard shoulder

The following parking procedure should be followed when you are the first emergency vehicle arriving at an unprotected scene on the hard shoulder:

- Stop 50 metres before the incident in a straight line with the carriageway.
- If there is no physical barrier or other obstruction, such as a bridge support, turn the front wheels towards the nearside; if there is a barrier, turn the front wheels outwards towards the carriageway. If the vehicle is subsequently struck from behind, it will then be steered away from you rather than pushed straight towards the incident you are attending.
- Switch off forward-facing blue lights and flashing headlights, but keep your rear-facing blue or red lights on (or both if fitted), as well as sidelights and hazard lights. Keeping the rear doors closed when possible will ensure that their reflective, high-visibility markings can be seen.
- If possible, stay behind the barrier when walking towards the incident. If this is not possible, stay as far away from the live carriageway as you can. Keep a lookout for approaching traffic.

Incidents on the main carriageway

If you are first on scene at an incident on the main carriageway, you may need to place your vehicle in a fend-off, fend-in or in-line position – refer to your local ambulance service's procedures.

These extremely hazardous positions involve using the vehicle to block one or more lanes, and should be performed with the utmost caution.

In-line vehicle positioning

With in-line positioning, the vehicle is parallel to the running lanes on the carriageway. This maximises rear-facing lighting and rear vehicle markings.

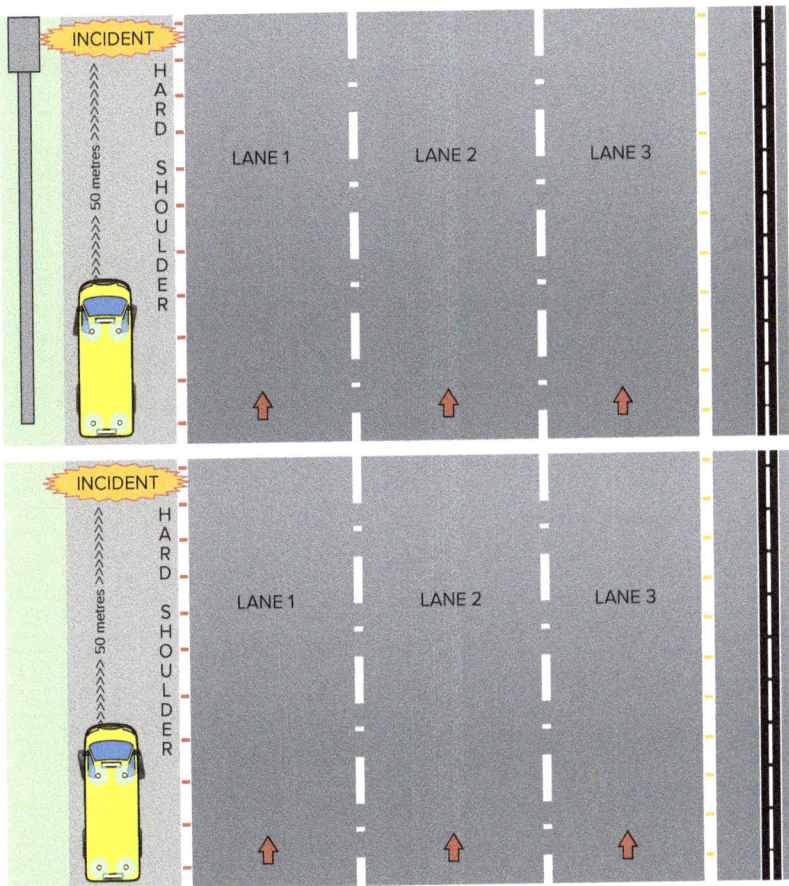

FIGURE 14.4 • In-line vehicle positioning for both with barrier (top) and without barrier (bottom).

Fend-in vehicle positioning

For fend-in positioning, the vehicle is angled, pointing front end towards the nearside in the direction the traffic should pass. This method fills the lane that is to be closed and acts as a visual reinforcement of the cone taper.

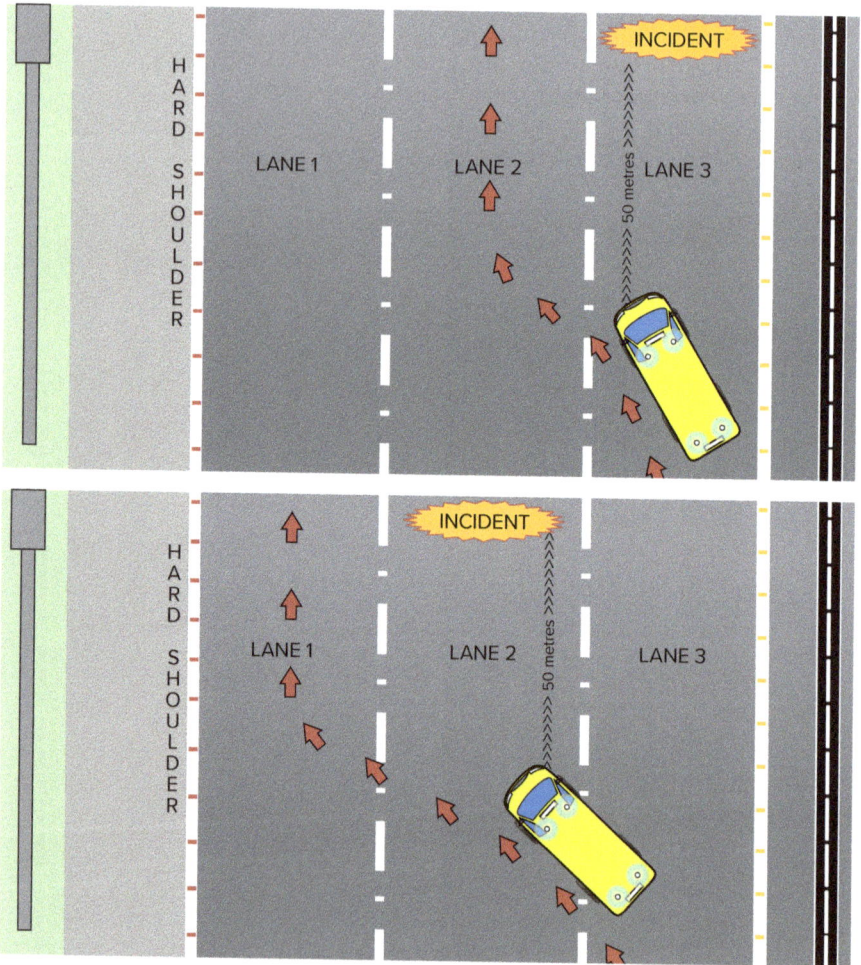

FIGURE 14.5 • Fend-in vehicle positioning from lane 3 (top) and lanes 2 and 3 (bottom).

Fend-off vehicle positioning

For fend-off positioning, the vehicle is angled, pointing front end towards the carriageway in the direction the traffic should pass. This method fills the lane that is going to be closed, and also acts as a visual reinforcement of the cone taper. It appears stationary to the approaching traffic.

On multi-lane carriageways on no account should the incident scene and responders form an island with traffic passing on both sides.

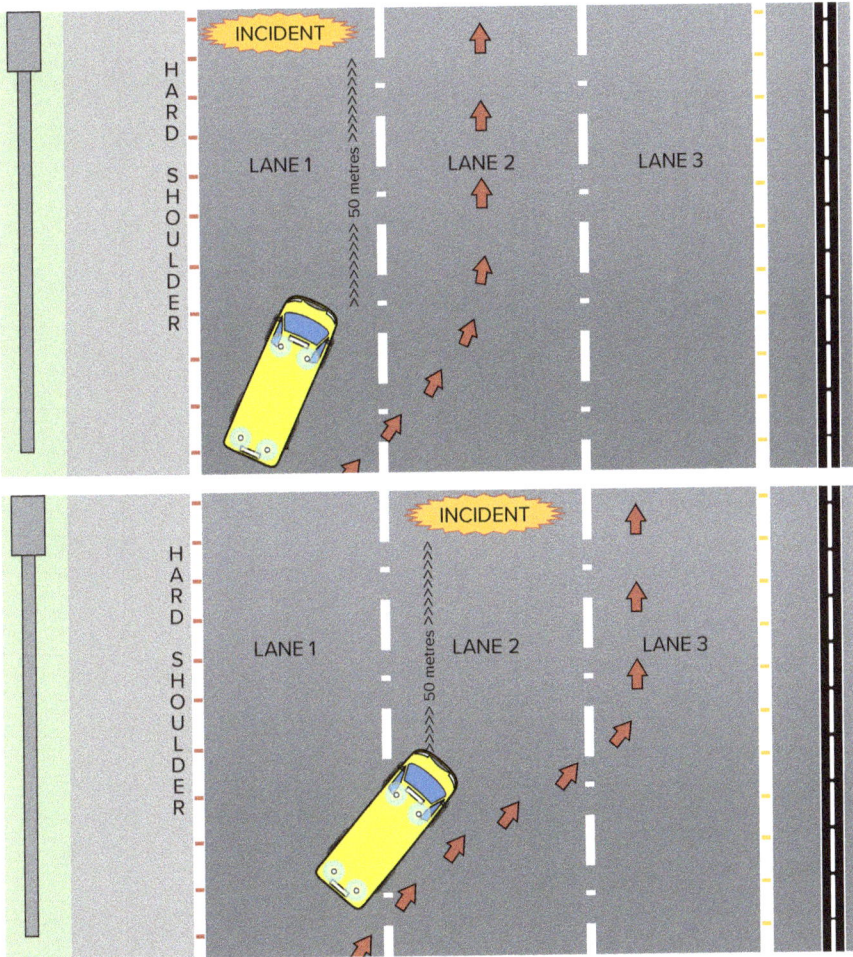

FIGURE 14.6 • Fend-off vehicle positioning in lane 1 (top) and in lanes 1 and 2 (bottom).

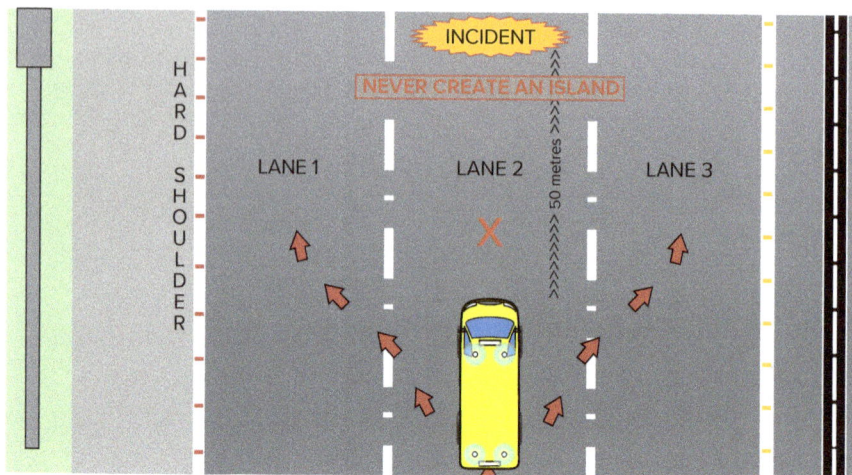

FIGURE 14.7 • Incorrect in-line vehicle positioning for multi-lane carriageways.

Leaving the Scene

Re-joining moving traffic when leaving the incident scene is also extremely hazardous – other road users may be too busy 'rubbernecking' to notice that you are moving.

If there is a clear path in front of you, you should proceed in a straight line in that lane or on the hard shoulder. You can change lanes when you have built up enough speed to match the traffic conditions around you. Your rear blue lights should remain activated until you have re-joined the normal traffic flow; you can then turn them off if not conveying patients to hospital as an emergency.

Situation Reports

If you are the first emergency vehicle on scene you should provide control with a situation report (SITREP) as soon as possible. A SITREP is a situation report provided to control, detailing your exact location, direction of travel, the number and types of vehicles involved in the incident, the number of casualties and whether further assistance is required. It should contain the following information:

- Your location – the nearest marker post (see Figure 14.8) will confirm your location to within 100 metres
- A driver location sign (see Figure 14.9) will give your position on motorways and some A roads (see below)

- Your direction of travel, for example northbound/southbound
- The number and types of vehicles involved in the incident
- Which lanes of the carriageway are involved
- Whether any hazardous loads are involved.

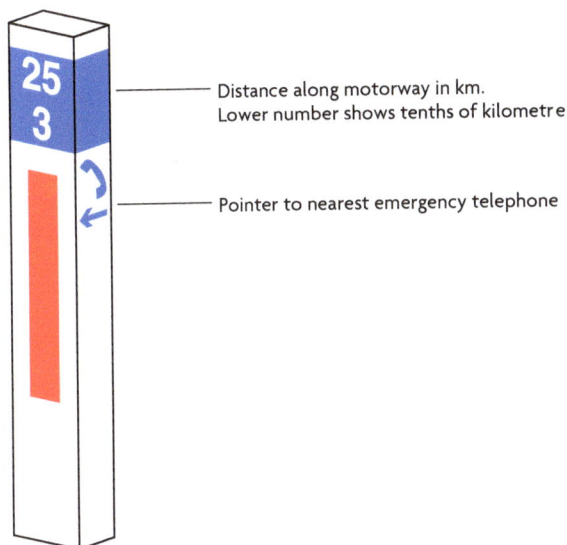

Distance along motorway in km.
Lower number shows tenths of kilometre

Pointer to nearest emergency telephone

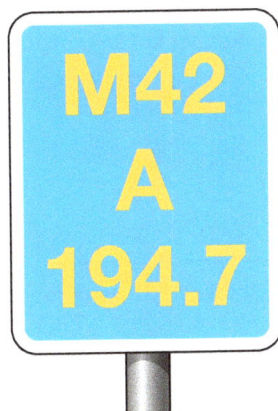

FIGURE 14.9 • Example of a driver location sign.

FIGURE 14.8 • Example of a marker post.

Marker posts are a distance in kilometres from a defined point and will give your location within 100 metres. The example post shown in Figure 14.8 is 25.3 km from the defined point.

This information will be passed on to the police or National Highways control – they will activate the matrix signs, if available, to warn approaching motorists.

Driver location signs are small and blue as shown in Figure 14.9. You will find them at the side of motorways, positioned every 500 metres, and on some major A roads.

Providing the details on the sign nearest to the incident will make it quicker for other agencies to find you.

- The top line shows which road you are on
- The letter on the second line – A or B – gives the direction in which you are travelling
- The bottom line tells you how far you are from a given location.

> ## ⓘ REMEMBER
>
> You must use the terms 'Lane 1', 'Lane 2' and 'Lane 3', not the 'slow lane', 'middle lane' or 'fast lane'.

You must keep control regularly informed. Subsequent SITREPs should include:

- The number of casualties
- The types of injuries sustained
- Requests for further vehicles if required
- Requests for air ambulance if required
- Whether assistance is required from other agencies, for example the fire and rescue service
- Notifying hospitals.

Other Urban and Rural Roads

Attending the scene of an incident on any road, including those in residential areas, presents a degree of risk. Emergency response crews should not become complacent and should be especially aware of the risks associated with 'red mist' – paying too much attention to what may be presented at the scene before arriving at it can allow intrusive thoughts to influence your decision-making process. Regardless of the medical competencies or skills the clinician may have, these hold no value until they have safely arrived at the scene.

As with motorways and dual carriageways, stopping on any high-speed road – or indeed anywhere where other vehicular activity is present – is potentially high risk, especially for covert vehicles that may be attending these incidents.

Non-emergency vehicles at scenes

Other vehicles that operate within organisations, for example PTS vehicles, may periodically come across incidents on highways and may not be fitted with the appropriate emergency warning equipment. In these instances, the driver should perform a dynamic risk assessment and consider whether it may be safer to park away from the incident and provide control with a situation report (see opposite) rather than to stop at the scene.

This can be very difficult, but you must not be tempted to put yourself in danger. See Appendix 1 for further information on non-emergency vehicles attending motorway or dual carriageway incidents.

Stopping and Parking at the Scene

When parking at the scene of any emergency, crew and vehicle safety must be paramount. Parking should, where possible, take place in an area that facilitates safe egress for staff, minimising the danger caused by passing vehicles.

Consideration should be given to the likelihood of patient loading, which would entail sufficient clearance required for ramps and tail lifts. If the vehicle is parked partly on the pavement, this may mean that the ramp or tail lift may not deploy correctly due to the kerb impeding its operation.

The use of warning lights should be appropriate for the density of hazards present or potentially present. In residential areas, the use of hazard warning lights alone may be sufficient, whereas other rural or urban roads may require the full use of emergency warning lighting.

When parking at night ensure that, as a minimum, the vehicle sidelights are illuminated, particularly if you have to park facing oncoming traffic.

Solo responders need to consider the most appropriate parking positions carefully, particularly in residential areas. Parking directly outside a private dwelling to attend to a patient may inconvenience any following back-up vehicle when they need to park and load a patient.

Consider:

- When approaching the scene ensure you maintain forward vision, anticipation and planning to facilitate a safe and controlled arrival.
- Park in a place that will facilitate safe egress for staff and minimise danger by passing vehicles.
- Park in a position that affords the maximum protection to crew, patient, other emergency services, helpers and bystanders at the scene.
- Consider patient loading i.e. access and space needed to operate the vehicle ramp.
- Emergency warning lights should be used if available on rural or urban roads to protect the scene.
- Consider deploying lookouts, wearing PPE, to warn oncoming traffic of the obstruction ahead.
- Perform continual Dynamic Risk Assessments as the environment is likely to evolve as the incident continues, consider what parking position offers max protection.
- PPE must always be put on prior to leaving the vehicle including hi-visibility jacket and helmet BOTH FASTENED.
- Consider unseen or unheard vehicles (blind spots).
- Consider what warning equipment is fitted that give you greater protection.
- Use passive protection to maximise safety, ie the visibility of the vehicle reflective panels in relation to the road layout.

- Parking 50 metres from the scene, as advised on motorways or dual carriageways, may not be possible or afford the best protection at the scene.
- A Dynamic Risk Assessment must be undertaken with due regard to the nature, environment and scale of the incident.
- Request police presence as early as possible to maintain safety and control passing traffic/road closures.
- The activation of rear red fashing lights is very effective due to their primary colour attraction; however, in the presence of mist or fog this can be distracting for other vehicles, which may not see you initially. Look, listen and be extremely vigilant about the potential of developing hazards as yet unseen.

ⓘ REMEMBER

While attending any incident, staff must consider the parking location carefully, not only for patient and crew access but, more importantly, whether it offers the maximum protection to other road users. Is there a safer alternative?

Your personal safety is paramount. It is vital that the correct use of PPE is adopted and that maximum visual warning is activated on the responding vehicle.

Police Escorts

Occasionally circumstances may dictate that an ambulance requires a police escort on its journey, for example if it is vital that the journey to hospital is a slow, uninterrupted and smooth one, or that the journey time is reduced. This request must usually be approved by ambulance control (refer to your local service's procedures). The police will provide an escort if they are in agreement that one will indeed cut the journey time or make it slower and safer, and if police resources are available.

The following procedure for escorts given by police motorcycles or other police vehicles has been offered by members of the Police Driver Standards Group:

- One motorcycle is positioned at the front of the ambulance, and it is its role to maintain a safe and constant speed.
- Another is positioned on the offside of the ambulance, visible in the ambulance's offside wing mirror.
- The final motorcycle is positioned to block off traffic at the next major hazard, such as a junction or a roundabout.
- As the ambulance goes through the hazard, the bike controlling the hazard takes up a position on the offside of the ambulance. The bike that was previously in this position moves up to control the next hazard.

Alternative procedures are in operation around the country, and it is in the interests of all services to work across boundaries and within written local policies and procedures.

There is no exemption available for the driver of an ambulance vehicle to claim exemption when escorting another vehicle to hospital. This is a specialised function and must only be completed by the police who do hold exemptions to do this.

(?) KNOWLEDGE RECAP

1. Explain why personal protective equipment is essential when attending incidents on a multi-lane carriageway.
2. What is 'scene preservation' and why is it important?
3. Which lanes should be used when approaching an incident on a motorway or dual carriageway in flowing traffic?
4. What precautions should be taken when approaching an incident on a motorway or dual carriageway by driving on the hard shoulder?
5. Explain the dangers of using sirens when responding in slow moving traffic on the hard shoulder of a motorway?
6. Why should a number of emergency vehicles responding to a single incident avoid travelling in a convoy?
7. Where is the correct place to park at an incident on a motorway or dual carriageway that is already being attended by another emergency service?
8. What are 'fend-off', 'fend-in' and 'in-line' parking positions and when would you use them?
9. What information should be relayed to control in a SITREP?
10. What information should be relayed to control in subsequent SITREPs?
11. Describe the procedure for leaving the scene of an incident on a motorway or dual carriageway, if the path ahead of you is clear.
12. What procedure should you follow if you come across an incident while driving a vehicle that is not fitted with emergency warning equipment?
13. In what circumstances might you request a police escort?
14. Can an ambulance solo responder provide an escort for another emergency ambulance vehicle in some circumstances?

CHAPTER 15

Smart Motorways

LEARNING OUTCOMES

By the end of this chapter you should:

- Understand the additional safety issues with responding to and attending incidents on the smart motorway network.
- Understand the process for reverse access and rearward relief.
- Understand the considerations for scene management on a smart motorway.

Smart motorways make use of a range of traffic management measures to control speeds, add capacity and inform road users of conditions on the network. These include:

- Variable mandatory speed limits (VMSLs) with associated enforcement and compliance system
- Driver information including lane availability, displayed at intervals not exceeding 1,500 metres – information is provided through a mixture of gantry- and verge-mounted signs and signals capable of displaying mandatory speed limits and full-carriageway mandatory lane closures
- Motorway service areas (MSAs) and other roadside facilities, which perform an important road safety function by providing road users with the opportunity to stop and take a break in the course of their journey
- Emergency roadside telephones (ERTs), which give a direct line to an operator
- Gantries with supporting variable message signs, sometimes also with signals, displaying automatically altered speed limits
- Motorway incident detection and automatic signalling (MIDAS) operating system.

Different Types of Smart Motorways

There are three types of smart motorways. The three types are listed below along with some of their key features:

All Lanes Running (ALR)

- No hard shoulder
- Emergency Refuge Areas (ERAs) coloured orange with emergency phone
- Stopped vehicle detection

Dynamic Hard Shoulder (DHS)

- Hard shoulder opened and closed depending on traffic flow/congestion
- Overhead electronic signs to inform when the hard shoulder can and cannot be used
- Motorway detection and automatic signalling (MIDAS)

Controlled Motorways

- Hard shoulder in place
- CCTV and enforcement cameras
- Overhead electronic signs to vary speed limits and open/close lanes

In 2023, the UK government stopped the rollout of any new smart motorways due to lack of public confidence and cost pressures.

Attending Incidents on Smart Motorways

Access via Normal Flow of Traffic on the Affected Carriageway

Emergency response in normal traffic flow will be the initial and preferred approach to attend incidents. This entails approaching the incident from the rear, using the carriageway on which the reported incident has occurred, and in the same direction as normal traffic flow.

Where traffic flows indicate that access can be achieved by travelling with the normal flow of traffic on the affected carriageway on an all-lane running motorway, the regional control centre (RCC) will set red 'X lane' closure signals to provide an access lane to the incident scene. This is because on an all-lane motorway, there is no hard shoulder for access. To encourage compliance, the red 'X's will be supplemented by the legend 'Lane closed for incident access' (see Figure 15.1).

The access lane will be established well in advance of the incident and can be set back as far as the previous junction, or beyond where necessary. Typically, the access lane will be established in Lane 1 for incidents occurring in nearside lanes and in Lane 4 for those occurring in offside lanes, as below:

- **Road traffic collision (RTC) in Lanes 1 and 2:** RCC will close Lane 1 to provide the access route
- **RTC in Lanes 3 and 4:** RCC will close Lane 4 to provide the access route
- **RTC in Lanes 2 and 3:** RCC will close Lane 1 to provide the access route (as first preference).

This approach aims to keep as many lanes as possible (from a safety point of view), open past the incident to keep traffic flowing and facilitate emergency response upstream on the affected carriageway. Note that while more than one lane may be closed at the incident scene, only one lane will be closed for incident access.

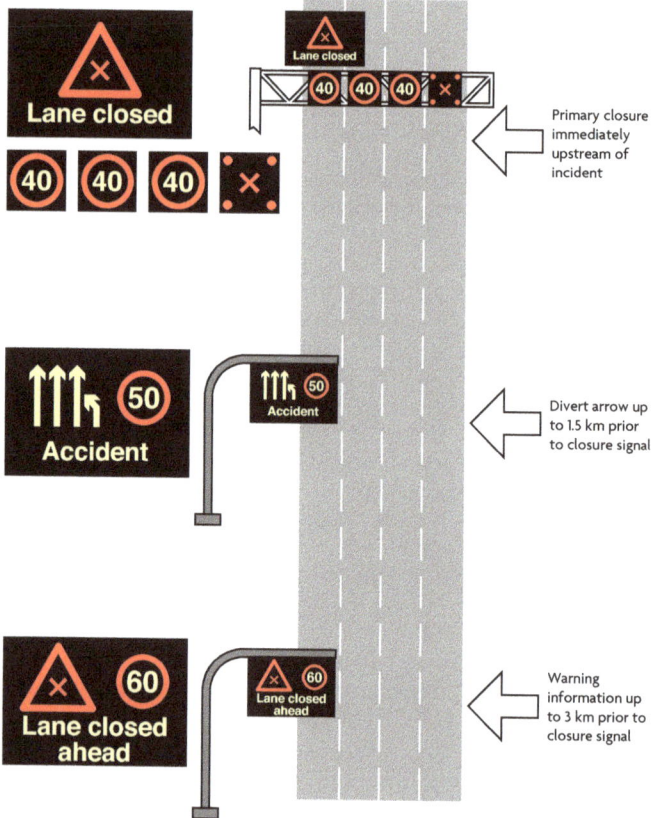

FIGURE 15.1 • Carriageway incident signalling.

Reverse Access

Using reverse access will normally be the tactical option in the early stages of an incident, when access with the flow of traffic on the affected carriageway becomes problematic for any reason.

Reverse access requires emergency vehicles to report to a rendezvous point (RVP) at the reverse flow access point (normally the next junction downstream from the incident). The personnel at the access point need to be instructed clearly on the procedure to be followed for reverse access, including turning safely into the carriageway at the end of the entry slip onto the motorway.

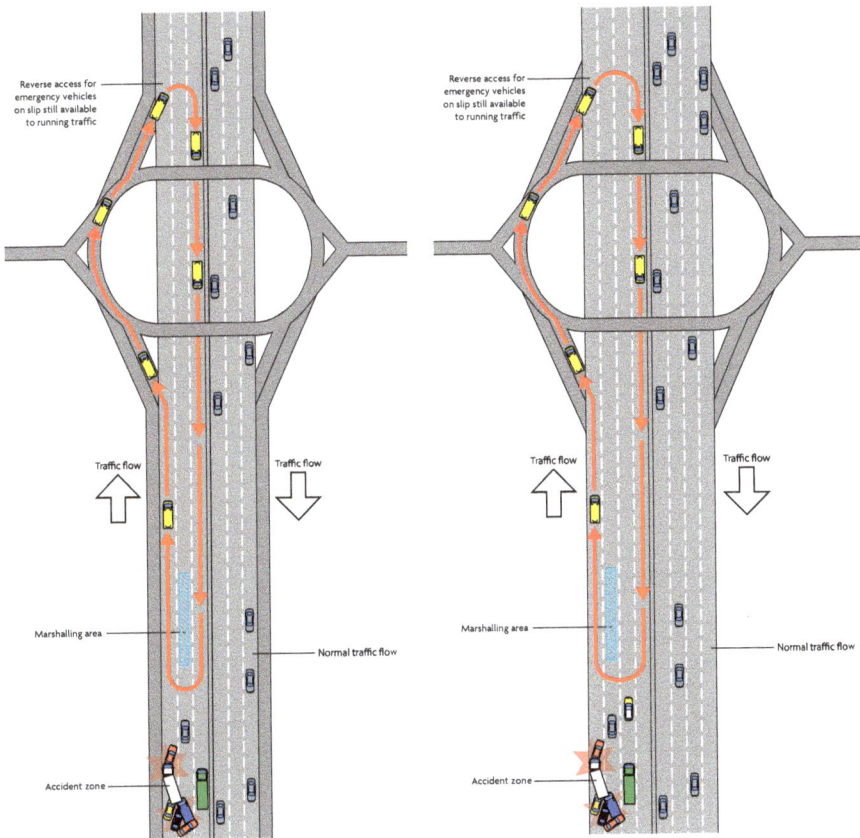

Reverse access for emergency vehicles on slip still available to running traffic

Reverse access for emergency vehicles on slip still available to running traffic

Traffic flow

Traffic flow

Traffic flow

Traffic flow

Marshalling area

Normal traffic flow

Marshalling area

Normal traffic flow

Accident zone

Accident zone

FIGURE 15.2 • Reverse access on a motorway with and without hard shoulder.

Emergency vehicles will enter the motorway on the 'on' slip road (except on junctions where there isn't an 'on' slip road in which case the 'off' slip road will be used) and turn right across the motorway to travel contraflow to the incident site. Caution should be exercised when crossing the carriageway at the entrance point as there may be vehicles passing along the carriageway in Lane 1.

Emergency vehicles will travel to the incident site in the offside lane (the lane nearest the central reserve) and leave the incident in the nearside lane, by the exit slip road. Emergency services vehicles accessing an incident using reverse access will be claiming an exemption from road traffic regulations.

Rearward Relief

Police and traffic officers may also use the same carriageway to release vehicles stuck behind an incident. This procedure is known as rearward relief and is solely the responsibility of the police and National Highways.

Opposite carriageway approaching

Approaching from the opposite carriageway will only be used in exceptional circumstances – it may be used to confirm that all traffic has been stopped on the reported carriageway, prior to instigating the reverse access procedure. In this circumstance, a double crewed police vehicle will access the opposite carriageway and, on approach to the scene, employ a rolling road block to bring all traffic to a halt. Once traffic has been stopped, the passenger in the police vehicle will get out of the vehicle, cross the central barrier and secure the scene by stopping all traffic. Once complete, the reverse access

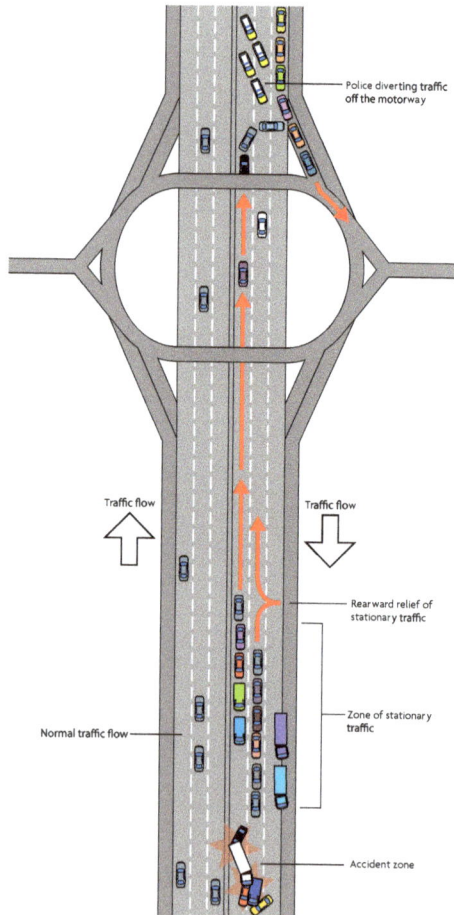

FIGURE 15.3 • Rearward relief.

procedure can be instigated and the police vehicle on the opposite carriageway will proceed and remove the rolling block.

Ambulance services and fire services cannot, under any circumstances, stop their vehicles on the opposite carriageway, unless the lane or carriageway is confirmed closed by the police or other appropriate organisations, such as National Highways or Transport Scotland's Trunk Road Incident Support Service (TRISS), and scene safety has been established.

Incident Scene Management

Management of the incident scene will begin when responders have reached the scene of operations and start undertaking scene safety duties. If in attendance, this is the responsibility of police or traffic officers, allowing other responders to focus on undertaking their core functions.

If police or traffic officers are not in attendance, the fire service will be responsible for scene safety and will adopt its own scene safety measures to protect operations and personnel at the scene.

Any lane closures and requests for variable message sign and signal changes made by the ambulance or fire service must be communicated to RCC via their respective control operators. This should also include a request for additional support from police and traffic officers as appropriate.

National Highways responsibility on scene is to enhance traffic management in accordance with the National Ambulance Resilience Unit's Guidance for Ambulance Service response to Incidents on the Motorway Network (Including Smart Motorways): 'Highways [...] will protect the scene by using signs and signals or by setting up emergency traffic management, enhanced traffic management or temporary traffic management and manage the outer cordon by placing interventions on the approach to the incident to manage traffic across motorway networks' (Department for Transport, 2009).

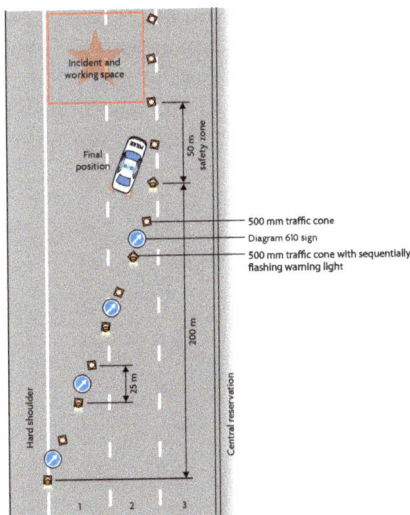

FIGURE 15.4 • Lanes 1 and 2 closed.

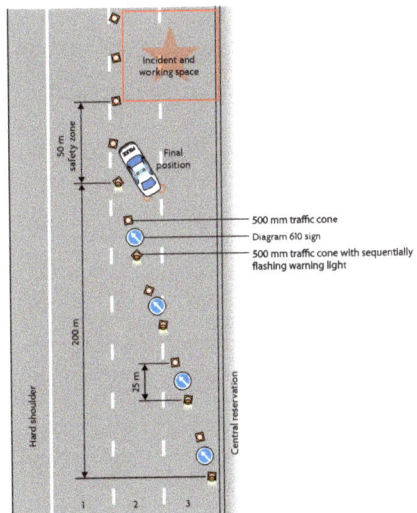

FIGURE 15.5 • Lanes 2 and 3 closed.

In the devolved nations, other organisations support the police in managing the flow of traffic on motorways and trunk roads. They may also assist in traffic management when incidents occur on these roads.

(?) KNOWLEDGE RECAP

1   What is an access lane and how will it be indicated?
2   What should you be particularly cautious of when undertaking reverse access on a smart motorway?
3   What is rearward relief used for?
4   Who can undertake opposite carriageway approaching?
5   Who is normally responsible for the scene on a smart motorway incident?

CHAPTER 16

Driving Commentary

LEARNING OUTCOMES

By the end of this chapter you should:

- Be able to identify the purpose of a driving commentary and the key skills in delivering an effective commentary.
- Understand how to give timely, relevant information when delivering a driving commentary.

Generally speaking, a commentary assists a driver to enhance their forward observation, planning and anticipation. Giving a commentary will allow you to concentrate on your drive and help to exclude intrusive and distracting thoughts. On driving courses, the commentary helps tutors to identify how far ahead the driver is observing hazards and assists in illustrating the thought process of a student. You can conduct a driving commentary when driving on your own or with others, in order to help you concentrate on the task of driving.

Any information provided by the driver should be current and not retrospective. The secret is to commence and complete the description well before the vehicle arrives at the subject of the commentary.

The content should, at times include quotes from *Roadcraft* and *The Highway Code* but this should not be to the detriment of more relevant subject matter existing at that time. Commentary during urban driving will provide little opportunity to include excerpts from *Roadcraft*, as there will invariably be a multitude of hazards to be concentrating on. In such environments there is so much occurring that the real art is to select the most appropriate hazard to discuss.

Rural driving presents different problems for the commentator. Speeds are higher, so the approach to the subject being discussed will provide less time for you to deliver any commentary. A common error on these types of roads is selecting an inappropriate subject matter, such as discussing principles of safe cornering on a straight section of road. The commentary must be relevant and any subject discussed needs to be at the correct time and location.

At first giving a commentary will appear very difficult, and you will feel self-conscious. A sound knowledge of *Roadcraft* and *The Highway Code* pays dividends and will assist in the development of a driver's commentary. Commentary skills should be developed in stages, initially concentrating on one subject, for example signs and lines, and then with each drive build up to other subjects, such as the weather, and then road surfaces.

An informative commentary should include a clear and early identification of hazards, the action that you intend to implement when approaching that hazard and the reason for that action, for example: 'Ahead I note there is a junction on the nearside with a restricted view into the mouth of that junction. I am therefore checking my mirrors and noting there are no opposing vehicles. I position my vehicle towards the crown of the road. I do this for three reasons: to provide me with a better view into the junction, to allow drivers using that junction to gain a view of my vehicle earlier and, finally, to allow a greater margin of safety on my vehicle's nearside should a vehicle overshoot the "give way" line.'

Introducing a Commentary

When commencing a commentary you should include the following information:

1   Type of vehicle you are driving
2   Type of road or environment
3   Speed limit applicable to that road or the vehicle you are driving
4   The prevailing weather and road surface conditions
5   Traffic density.

Examples of Introductions to Commentaries

'I am driving an ambulance response car on a two-lane single undivided carriageway in a rural environment, which is subject to the national speed limit of 60 mph. The weather is sunny, visibility is good and the road surface is dry and in good condition. Traffic flow is light.'

'I am driving a Mercedes Sprinter ambulance on a two-lane single undivided carriageway in an urban environment, which is subject to a 30 mph speed limit. The weather is dull with spells of rain, which has reduced my visibility, and the road surface is damp. Traffic flow is heavy.'

'I am driving a Mercedes Sprinter ambulance on a two-lane dual carriageway in a rural environment. The road is subject to the national speed limit of 70 mph, however my class of vehicle has a speed limit of 60 mph. The weather is dry but cold and the road surface is slippery. Traffic flow is currently moderate to heavy.'

Observation Links

Drivers should at all times try to notice even small details, as this can provide valuable and early information that allows the driver to predict or anticipate the presence of danger or likely actions of other road users. A driver should constantly aim to build up a stock of observation links. It enhances a driver's air of professionalism when a driver predicts an occurrence for it then to happen as predicted. Some observations links are shown below, but this is obviously not an exhaustive list.

- **Skid marks:** indicate areas of danger where other drivers have experienced issues.
- **Dustbins at the side of the road:** indicate the presence of refuse collection lorry – the refuse collection lorry could be on your side of the road travelling towards you and the operatives could be crossing the road.
- **Following a bus:** look into the vehicle to establish whether passengers are standing up, which may result in the bus stopping; also looking ahead of the vehicle to search for bus stops where people may be waiting to catch the bus.

- **Stationary bus:** expect it to suddenly pull away, pedestrians to walk from beyond the front or rear of the bus to cross the road, or somebody running across road to catch the bus.
- **Sunlight/shadows at gateways, private entrances or junctions:** the absence of shadows indicates an absence of vehicles/pedestrians.
- **Reflections:** utilise shop windows, vehicle glass and paintwork to see around corners.
- **Tyre noise:** a good rule of thumb on tarmac surfaces is – the more noise being generated by the tyre/road interface the better the grip.
- **Smell of grass cuttings:** possible workers or works vehicles in the vicinity cutting the verges/hedges.
- **Microclimates:** pay attention to shaded areas under trees, for example, where dampness or ice may linger.
- **Work vehicles:** the presence of one work vehicle may indicate another work vehicle is nearby.
- **Person up a telegraph pole:** their van will be nearby.
- **Field gates open:** is there a tractor or farm animals on the road?
- **Marker posts at the side of the road:** a hazard to either the left or right. White reflectors on the top of the post indicate the road is bending to the left or there is a hazard to the left, red reflectors mean the road is bending to the right or there is a hazard to the right. Examples of hazards may be concealed entrances/exits, turning points, gated fields or concealed roads.
- **Traffic turning ahead:** other vehicles may follow or emerge.
- **White line systems:** the more paint the more danger – but solid double white lines, where the line nearest to you is broken, may present an overtaking opportunity.
- **Pedal cycles:** prone to wobbling and affected by cross winds; an over-shoulder glance may precede a change of direction.
- **Mud on the road:** affects road holding and handling – its presence could also indicate the likelihood of agricultural vehicles in the vicinity.
- **Post Office vans:** where is the driver? Could they be about to alight or return to vehicle?
- **Lay-bys:** could a vehicle emerge? Could a vehicle enter the lay-by slowly or with little advanced warning? A person could be exercising a dog.
- **'Slow' painted on road:** if painted prior to a bend, there will be an associated danger i.e. private entrance, lay-by, field entrance, junction, bend or adverse camber.
- **Animal droppings:** where is the animal that deposited the droppings?
- **Dead leaves:** can be very slippery, particularly when wet (hence the ability of 'leaves on the line' to disrupt entire rail networks), and may be hiding pot holes in the road.

- **Farm buildings:** possible agricultural vehicles nearby, possible mud on the road, possible livestock movement.
- **Tractors:** could move into field entrances – be aware of suspended implements and the fact that they may not possess indicators, so the driver may have to use hand signals.
- **Telegraph poles:** can sometimes indicate the path of the road, however be aware they do not always follow the path of the road.
- **Lamp posts:** very good indicators of the path of road, however, be aware that those in the distance may be associated with a side road or estate. A single or small group of lamp posts can locate junctions on motorways, as well as on rural or urban roads. Lamp posts forming a circle indicate the position of a roundabout.
- **Unofficial road signs:** sometimes more relevant than those placed by local authorities as they probably are current, e.g. 'car boot sale' or 'tractors turning'.
- **Traffic signs:** all should be described accurately:

  Observe
  Understand
  React

  Where road signs are stacked (two or three together) the uppermost sign will be the first hazard you will encounter.
- **Brake lights ahead:** check mirrors as there could be hazards ahead.
- **Zebra crossing:** watch for pedestrians approaching, look for rearward glances as this is normally a sign that they are about to use the crossing.
- **Pelican, puffin or toucan crossing:** look for pedestrians pushing the button mounted on the control box, which will eventually cause the traffic lights to change to red.
- **Village nameplate:** you are about to enter a speed limit and there is likely to be an increase in hazards.
- **Strike kerbs:** provide protection to pavements by discouraging drivers to mount their near vertical face.
- **Puddles:** could be deep and hide large unseen objects.
- **Convex mirrors:** mounted on the sides of a road to assist drivers to enter the main road from concealed entrances.
- **Phone boxes:** could somebody be rushing to make that once-in-a-lifetime call?
- **Edge of carriageway markings:** denotes the side of the road; where broken this indicates private drives, field entrances etc.
- **Dogs on leads:** identify whether or not they are restrained. What is the size differential between the dog and the person? Is the dog reacting to the presence of the vehicle?
- **Emergency vehicles on calls:** are other similar vehicles approaching?
- **Muddy tyre tracks:** where is the tractor or other vehicle that caused them?

- **Dropped kerb:** dropped kerbs allow pedestrians with bikes and wheelchairs to access crossing points, while also allowing vehicles into parking places.
- **LGV approaching incline:** anticipate speed reduction.
- **Is the LGV laden/unladen?** Look for the amount of tyre bulge and suspension 'bounce'.
- **Cross winds:** look for foliage moving, discuss how other vehicles may be affected, or how your vehicle may respond to those cross winds.
- **Spray being thrown up by other vehicles:** locates water on road – check for excess surface water and anticipate that vehicles ahead may brake suddenly, to avoid aquaplaning remember to lose speed (by deceleration in the first instance).
- **Wet tyre marks on other side of the road:** expect water ahead; similarly if oncoming vehicles are using headlights and look wet, anticipate rainy weather ahead.
- **Factory premises:** expect movement of LGVs or forklift trucks.
- **'Give way' signs:** note that these are inverted triangles – stop signs are octagonal.
- **Learner drivers:** could stall as they move off from stationary.
- **Foreign registered vehicles:** may carry out unorthodox manoeuvres.
- **Hire vehicles:** may be unfamiliar to the driver.

Commentary on the System

It is important that you learn the phases of the system of car control and put them into operation. Try doing this for hazards such as traffic lights, major junctions, obstructions and where you intend to turn. Now you have to fill in the spaces between the systems, and for this you need a good knowledge of *The Highway Code*.

Roadcraft defines the system of car control thus:

> 'The system of car control is a way of approaching and negotiating hazards that is methodical, safe and leaves nothing to chance. It involves careful observation, early anticipation and planning, and a systematic use of the controls to maintain your vehicle's stability in all situations. The system consists of processing information and four phases – position, speed, gear and acceleration. Each phase develops out of the one before.'

Police Foundation, 2020

A hazard is anything that is an actual or potential danger. When providing a commentary, the system should be described accurately. Below is an example of a left turn from a major road into a minor nearside road:

> 'Processing information: I can see the nearside junction ahead, into which I intend to turn left.

I conduct mirror checks and, in the absence of nearside dangers, I position the vehicle to the nearside about half a metre from the verge. Position is now correct.

I conduct further mirror checks and then apply the left indicator. I then reduce speed by application of the footbrake (or by acceleration sense). My aim is to have achieved the correct speed about three vehicle lengths from the junction. Speed is correct.

I now select second gear, which is the correct gear for the speed. I conduct final mirror checks prior to applying the correct degree of acceleration to negotiate and leave the hazard safely.'

Spot Commentary

Spot commentaries are used to highlight particular aspects of driving. The next few sections suggest areas that you may wish to include in your commentary, where relevant.

Acceleration Sense

The term 'acceleration sense' is used by emergency response drivers to mean the ability to vary a vehicle's speed according to changing road and traffic conditions using the accelerator alone, meaning less use of braking (Police Foundation, 2020). Consider how you might include examples of acceleration sense in a commentary.

Types of Hazard

It's useful to think in terms of three types of hazard:

- Physical features (e.g. junctions, bends, road surface)
- The position or movement of other road users (e.g. drivers, cyclists, pedestrians)
- Weather conditions (e.g. icy road, poor visibility).

There are likely to be multiple examples of each type of the first two hazards for you to include in a commentary on most journeys.

Safe Cornering

The key principles of safe cornering are as follows.

1 Make sure that your vehicle is in the correct position on the approach.
2 Travel at the correct speed for the corner or bend.
3 Select the correct gear for that speed.

4   Use the accelerator to maintain a constant speed through the bend.

5   Be able to stop safely within the distance you can see to be clear on your own side of the road.

Here is an example of commentary on cornering:

> *'Ahead I note there is a gradual right bend. I conduct mirror checks and in the absence of any nearside dangers I position the vehicle close to the nearside, approximately half a metre from the verge. I do this to improve my safety, view and stability. By using limit point analysis, and having checked the mirrors, I will adjust the speed of the vehicle. Now that the speed is right I will select second gear, which is correct for this speed. After checking the mirrors, I will apply the accelerator to ensure I maintain a constant speed to negotiate and leave the bend safely. My speed is such that I can stop the vehicle safely within the distance I can see to be clear on my own side of the road.'*

Limit Point

The limit point is the furthest point of which you have an uninterrupted view of the road surface. Try to include terms like this in your commentary.

Following Position

Keeping your distance increases your safety because:

* You have a good view, and can increase it along both sides – this enables you to be fully aware of what is happening on the road ahead.
* You can stop your vehicle safely if the driver in front brakes firmly without warning.
* You can extend your braking distance so that the driver behind has more time to react, especially if they are driving too close.
* You can see when it's safe to move into the overtaking position.
* In wet weather, spray from the vehicle in front is reduced.

(?) KNOWLEDGE RECAP

1   How can a driving commentary help you to focus on the task of driving?
2   Why does a commentary help during driver training or development?
3   How should you start your commentary?
4   Why are observational links particularly useful?
5   What are the advantages of talking about the system of car control during your commentary?

Appendices

Appendix 1: Patient Transport and Unmarked Vehicles Attending Incidents on the Road Network (Including Fast Roads)

A fast road is classed as any road with a speed limit in excess of 40 mph.

Patient Transport staff and those driving unmarked vehicles must not attend incidents on the road network without the correct personal protective equipment (PPE). Service policy must be followed for the exact clothing and safety equipment to be worn when working on or near the road.

In broad terms, all staff should wear a high-visibility jacket (zipped up), safety boots and, in some cases, a protective safety helmet.

High Dependency Service (HDS) Vehicles

HDS vehicles should only be sent to an incident on a fast road, motorway or multi-lane carriageway if the presence of a safe coned-off area has been confirmed; they should park within this coned area following the same arrangements as other emergency vehicles.

HDS vehicles must not be used in fend-off positions if they are not fitted with appropriate visibility markings and adequate emergency warning lights – refer to your local service policy.

Patient Transport Service (PTS) Vehicles

PTS vehicles should only attend incidents on a fast road, motorway or multi-lane carriageway if it has been closed or a safe coned-off area has been confirmed. They should then follow the same parking arrangements as other emergency and utility vehicles.

Like HDS vehicles, PTS vehicles must not be used in fend-off positions if they do not have adequate emergency warning lights and appropriate high-visibility markings.

Unmarked Vehicles

Unmarked vehicles should park in the coned-off area, towards the front, making sure that they do not block the exit of other emergency vehicles.

They should not be used in fend-off positions except where organisational policy allows this to be undertaken.

Patient Transport, CFRs and Unmarked Cars Arriving First at Scene

Using unmarked vehicles to provide protection from other traffic on fast road networks can be very dangerous, even if those vehicles are fitted with emergency warning equipment.

Drivers of these vehicles should conduct a full risk assessment when arriving at an unprotected scene and comply with their local organisational policies and procedures to ensure their safety.

If you arrive first at the scene of an incident in an unmarked vehicle generally you should:

1 Perform a dynamic risk assessment – if the situation is unsafe, do not stop and report the incident to the control centre.

2 Switch on any visual warning devices available.

3 Park in a position that affords maximum safety to the crew and any patients on board.

4 Contact the control centre with an initial SITREP.

Do not, in any case, be tempted to put yourself in danger.

Appendix 2: Traffic Officers

Traffic officers operate on the Strategic Road Network (SRN), mainly motorways. They have powers to:

* Stop vehicles, or
* Make them proceed in, or keep to, a particular line of traffic.

They exercise these powers at incident scenes to:

* Maintain or improve the movement of traffic
* Prevent or reduce the effect of anything causing (or which has the potential to cause) congestion or other disruption to the movement of traffic
* Avoid danger to persons or other traffic (or prevent risks of any such danger arising)
* Prevent damage to, or to anything on or near a road they operate on.

Traffic officers will lead in the management of incidents in which there is no injury or alleged offences, using their powers to:

- Deal with congestion
- Ensure the safe and speedy removal of obstructions
- Assist vulnerable road users.

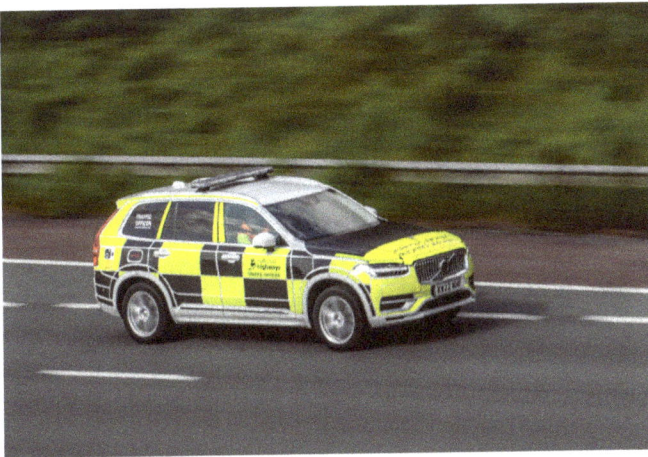

FIGURE A2.1 • Traffic officer vehicle.

The police will maintain scene control for any incidents that involve:

- Death
- Injury
- Criminality
- Threats to public order and safety
- Major coordination of emergency responders.

Powers Granted to Traffic Officers

Traffic officers' powers are detailed in the **Traffic Management Act 2004**. As well as having their own defined powers, as shown above, Section 4 sets out the legal relationship between Traffic officers and the police, and states that:

- When carrying out their duties a traffic officer shall comply with any direction of a police officer.
- Subject to that, when carrying out their duties a traffic officer when designated by an authorised person, shall comply with any direction of the appropriate national authority.

Ambulance staff should note that traffic officers' powers are restricted. They are trained to deal with incidents on the SRN and in order carry out their duty they may:

- Stop or direct traffic, including cyclists and, where necessary, implement rolling road blocks
- Place temporary traffic signs (emergency traffic management)
- Direct persons on foot
- Liaise with other responders and Maintenance Service Providers (MSP) who are contracted by National Highways to maintain the network.

On the arrival of ambulance staff, traffic officers will look to give an update on the number, age, gender and injuries of the casualties. They will also ask if any further safety measures are required, such as additional lane closures.

Traffic officers have a responsibility to inform the ambulance regional control centres for strategic roads and will need to know the number of casualties requiring treatment and what hospital they will be taken to. A basic state of injury will also be required.

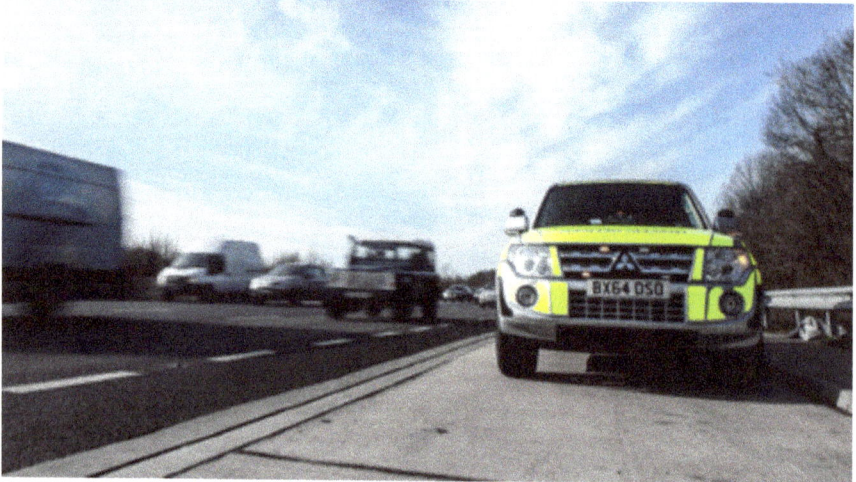

FIGURE A2.2 • Traffic officer vehicles operate on strategic road networks such as motorways.

Driver First Assist Training

Traffic officers are often first on the scene to help when drivers are in trouble; for this reason they receive Driver First Assist training on how to implement the recovery position and CPR, respond to a cardiac arrest and shock, and treat wounds and bleeding. Once the incident scene is safe, traffic officers can then put the nationally recognised Driver First Assist training into practice. The training has been made specific to the environment traffic officers work in, and allows them to provide direct assistance that can save lives in the crucial few minutes before the emergency services arrive.

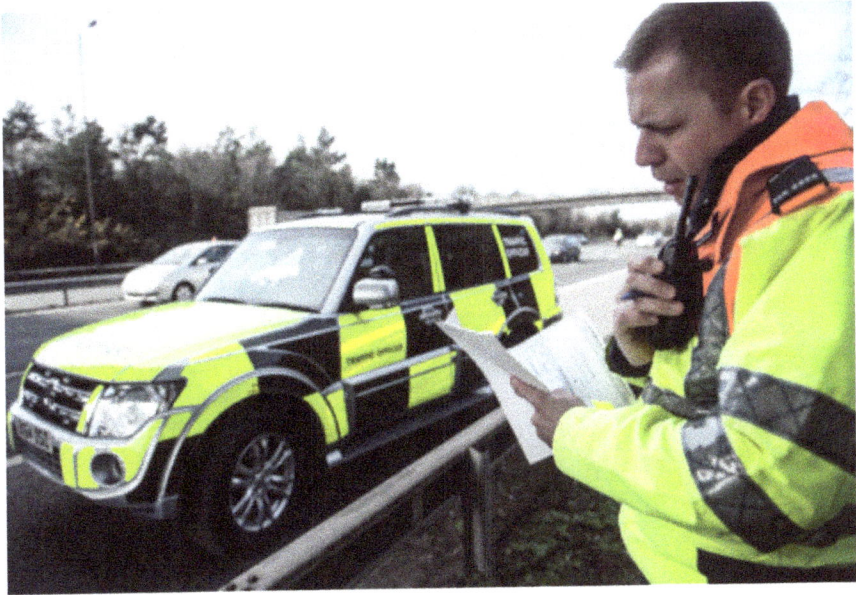

FIGURE A2.3 • Traffic Officer.

Appendix 3: Speed and Safety

The following is a talk by Mr Justice Blair outlining his 'Feet per Second' theory recorded in the *Journal of Criminal Law* in 1988:

> The basic cause of road accidents is widespread ignorance of ground speed, not only on the part of pedestrians but also on the part of virtually every driver of a motorcar, and I add that if this widespread ignorance on the part of the road users be cured, and it is curable, then there will follow a great reduction in the toll of road accidents.

> A speedometer does not tell anyone his ground speed. It does nothing of the kind, and it is because every motorist deludes himself into believing that a speedometer tells him how fast he is covering the ground that the danger of road accidents is increased. A speedometer gives you your speed in miles per hour. Have you any mental picture of the length of any hour or the length of a mile? No one has. How then can anyone possibly

get a mental picture of his ground speed when he is asked to put two unreliable factors together and obtain a result?

I have tried very many running down cases. Judges are conscientious when trying cases and I always felt that in order to understand any motor case it was necessary that I work out a respective speed of each vehicle in a measure that would tell me their respective ground speeds. The only measure that would give me any mental picture of the speed at which a vehicle covered the ground was the measure of feet per second. That involved me in a lot of arithmetic. Sixty miles per hour works out at 87.9 recurring feet per second, and every time I converted miles per hour into feet per second I got a result in recurring decimals. So then I had to look for a simple formula, and this is how I got it.

Instead of calling 60 miles per hour 87 odd feet per second, I called it 90 feet per second, and that gave me the simple formula of adding half to my miles per hour to obtain speed in feet per second correct within two per cent. Ever since then, I have driven cars and tried running down cases in feet per second. Now what I say to all motorists is that they try doing what I do; that is, always to drive and think of speed in feet per second instead of in miles per hour, and you will at once become a 100 per cent better and safer driver. All you have to do is to add one half to the figure of your speed in miles per hour and you will get your speed in feet per second.

Any child can do that. The other aspect of road safety touches what is called kinetic energy, which means the moving force possessed by a vehicle in motion. I can't give you a more detailed explanation but another way to put it is to refer to kinetic energy as the kick possessed by a moving vehicle. A small motor car weighing about a ton and moving at a speed of 40 miles per hour strikes the same blow as 18 ten-ton steamrollers travelling at their highest speed, which is 3 miles per hour. That is the force you are handling when you speed a light car up to 40 miles per hour, 60 feet per second. If you are driving a big seven-seater, two-ton car at 60 miles per hour (90 feet per second) its kinetic energy is more than that of 100 ten-ton steam rollers moving at 3 miles per hour.

Unhappily, human nature is such that, when travelling from one place to another, drivers are all inspired with the same desire: to get to a destination as soon as possible, travelling as fast as possible, the controls comprised by the words 'possible' being:

1 Regard for your safety
2 Road sense
3 Consideration for others
4 The law.

Consideration of 'feet per second' and 'kinetic energy' (see Table A3.1) do not occur to most of us until after an accident.

TABLE A3.1   Justice Blair's theory.

Feet per sec	Metres per sec	Miles per hour	Multiplier	Braking distance		Thinking distance		Overall stopping	
				Feet	Metres	Feet	Metres	Feet	Metres
45	13.73	30	1.5	45	13.73	30	9.15	75	22.88
60	18.30	40	2	80	24.40	40	12.20	118	36.60
75	22.88	50	2.5	125	38.13	50	15.25	175	53.38
90	27.45	60	3	180	54.90	60	18.30	240	73.20
105	32.03	70	3.5	245	74.73	70	21.35	315	96.08
120	36.60	80	4	320	97.60	80	24.40	400	122.00
135	41.18	90	4.5	405	123.53	90	27.45	495	150.98
150	45.75	100	5	500	152.50	100	30.50	600	183.00
165	50.33	110	5.5	605	184.53	110	33.55	715	218.08
180	54.90	120	6	720	219.60	120	36.60	840	256.20
195	59.48	130	6.5	845	257.73	130	39.65	975	297.38
210	64.05	140	7	980	298.90	140	42.70	1120	341.60
225	68.73	150	7.5	1125	343.13	150	45.75	1275	388.88
240	73.20	160	8	1280	390.40	160	48.80	1440	439.20
255	77.78	170	8.5	1445	440.73	170	51.85	1615	492.58
270	82.35	180	9	1620	494.10	180	54.90	1800	549.00
285	86.93	190	9.5	1805	550.53	190	57.95	1995	608.48
300	91.50	200	10	2000	610.00	200	61.00	2200	671.00

Appendix 4: Vehicle Fires

Vehicle fires are extremely rare with the modern vehicle engineering however, if your vehicle catches fire or start to issue smoke you should follow the below steps.

- Stay calm and don't panic
- Activate hazards and/or emergency lights
- Stop the vehicle is the safest possible place in the shortest time possible
- Turn your wheels to the direction of least risk in the event that the brakes fail once parked
- Apply the handbrake and turn off the ignition
- Get everyone away from the vehicle to a safe place preferably upwind and behind hard cover
- If normal exits are not accessible e.g. due to a collision use an emergency exit
- If you have a patient on board with limited mobility, make every possible attempt by whichever means to extricate them as long as you can keep yourself safe, consideration should be given to in-vehicle fire extinguishers to aid your escape, but you should familiarise yourselves on whether the type of extinguisher is safe to use in a confined space

- Once in a safe place make yourselves as visible as possible e.g. wearing hi-vis clothing and helmet
- Call 999 or 112 and ask for fire, tell them as much information as possible (M)ETHANE
  - Exact location – consider what 3 words
  - Type of incident – electric vehicle fire or Internal Combustion Engine fire
  - Hazards – large oxygen cylinders on board
  - Access/Egress – the road maybe obstructed so providing detailed instructions is key
  - Number of casualties – is anyone still trapped or injured
  - Emergency services present and requires
- Your regional EOC should also be informed via handheld radio or telephone providing the same information as above
- Do not return to the vehicle to collect any belongings.

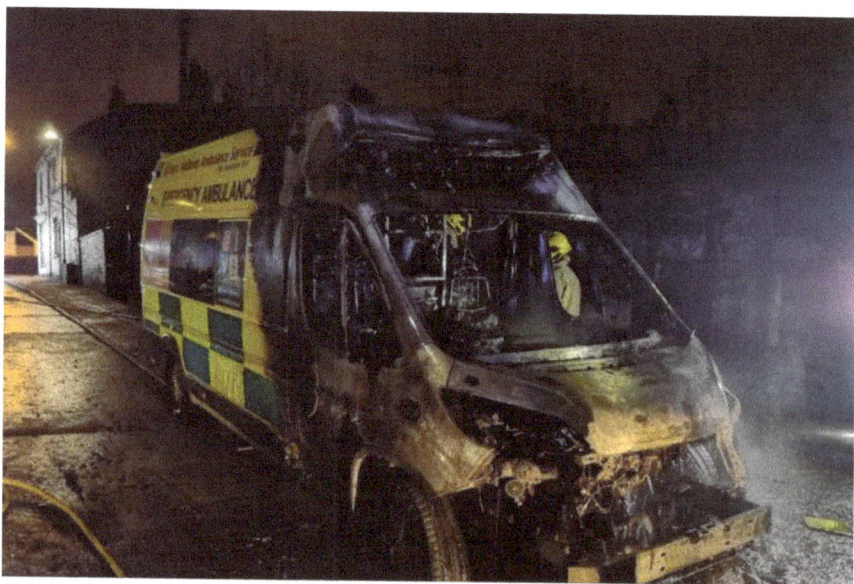

FIGURE A4.1 • Vehicle fire.

Appendix 5: Goals for Driver Education

Levels of Driver Behaviour	Essential Elements of Driver Training		
	Knowledge and Skills to Master	Awareness of Risk-Increasing Factors	Self-Evaluation
Level 1 Vehicle Control and Manoeuvring	Knowledge and skills concerning: • control of direction and position • tyre grip and friction • technical aspects of vehicle • physical handling when cornering, accelerating and braking	Risks associated with: • insufficient skills • poor speed adjustment • difficult road conditions • improper use of seat belt, head restraint, etc. • under-inflated or worn tyres	Self-evaluation and awareness of: • understanding of essential knowledge and skills • strengths and weaknesses of basic vehicle control • ability to control the vehicle in challenging conditions
Level 2 Mastery of Traffic Situations	Knowledge and skills concerning: • traffic rules • observation • signals • anticipation • speed adjustment • safety margins	Risks caused by: • wrong expectations/ assumptions • vulnerable road users • disobeying rules • unpredictable behaviour • information overload • difficult conditions such as darkness	Self-evaluation and awareness of: • ability to deal with a variety of traffic situations • observational skills • planning and anticipation • personal driving style • personal safety margins
Level 3 Goals and Context of Driving	Knowledge and skills concerning: • purpose of the journey • route planning • evaluation of required driving time • evaluation of necessity of journey • safety and control of passengers	Risks connected with: • driver's physiological condition • purpose of the journey • driving environment such as rural/urban or day/night • social context and in-vehicle company	Self-evaluation and awareness of: • own physiological condition • journey planning skills • typical journey goals or expectations • typical risky driving motives • self-critical thinking skills

(Continued)

Essential Elements of Driver Training			
Levels of Driver Behaviour	Knowledge and Skills to Master	Awareness of Risk-Increasing Factors	Self-Evaluation
Level 4 Personal Goals for Life and Skills for Living	Knowledge of and control over: • how life goals and personal tendencies affect driving behaviour • personal motives and competencies • lifestyle/life situation • age-related issues • personal values and ambitions	Risks related to: • acceptance of risk • self-enhancement through driving • high sensation seeking • susceptibility to social pressure • use of alcohol or drugs • personal values and attitudes to society	Self-evaluation and awareness of: • personal skills for impulse control • attitude towards risk • introspective competence • risky tendencies and habits • safety-negative motives
Level 5 Social Environment	Knowledge of and control over: • cultural and sub-cultural issues • work-related issues • group goals, values and motives • social environment and position	Risks related to: • cultural or work issues impacting on driving • context of journey such as work or pleasure • passengers	Self-evaluation and awareness of: • how culture or work issues impact on driving decisions and judgements • how placement within social group or work environment influences choices

Source: Based on the work of Hatakka et al. (2002) and Keskinen et al. (2010).

List of Abbreviations

AACE	Association of Ambulance Chief Executives
ABS	Antilock Brake System
ALR	All Lanes Running
ASR	Acceleration Skid Control
BAS	Brake Assist System
BASICS	British Association for Immediate Care Schemes
CFR	Community First Responder
COP	Codes of Practice
DHS	Dynamic Hard Shoulder
DTAG	Driver Training Advisory Group
DVLA	Driver and Vehicle Licensing Agency
EBA	Emergency Brake Assist
EBD	Electronic Brakeforce Distribution
ERA	Emergency Refuge Area
ERD	Emergency Response Driving
ERT	Emergency Roadside Telephones
ESC	Electronic Stability Control
ESP	Electronic Stability Programme
EV	Electric Vehicle
EWE	Emergency Warning Equipment
GPS	Global Positioning System
HART	Hazardous Area Response Team
HDS	High-Dependency Service
HSDT	High Speed Driving Training
LEZ	Low Emission Zone

LGV	Large Goods Vehicle
MIDAS	Motorway Incident Detection and Automatic Signalling
MSA	Motorway Service Areas
MSP	Maintenance Service Providers
PCV	Passenger Carrying Vehicle
PDC	Pre-Driving Check
PPE	Personal Protective Equipment
PTS	Patient Transport Service
RCC	Regional Control Centre
RDS	Radio Data System
RTC	Road Traffic Collision
RVP	Rendezvous Point
SITREP	Situation Report
SRN	Strategic Road Network
TRISS	Trunk Road Incident Support Service
TRO	Traffic Regulation Order
VDI	Vehicle Daily Inspection
VMSL	Variable Mandatory Speed Limits

References

AA (2017) Drive smart and save: How to get more out of the fuel you buy. Available at: http://www.theaa.com/driving-advice/fuels-environment/drive-smart [Accessed: May 2025].

Blair, Justice, 'Think in Feet Per Second', *The Benalla Standard*. 22 March 1938. Available at: https://trove.nla.gov.au/newspaper/article/269689661. Also reported in *Journal of Criminal Law* (1988), 52: https://journals.sagepub.com/toc/clja/52/3.

Department for Transport (2009) *Traffic Signs Manual – Chapter 8: Traffic Safety Measures and Signs for Road Works and Temporary Situations* (Part 2: Operations). London: The Stationery Office.

Department for Transport (2022) Smart Motorway Comparison Report. Available at: https://www.gov.uk/government/publications/smart-motorway-comparison-report-december-2022/smart-motorway-comparison-report-december-2022 [Accessed: March 2025].

Department for Transport (2023) All new smart motorways scrapped. Available at: https://www.gov.uk/government/news/all-new-smart-motorways-scrapped [Accessed: March 2025].

Dorn L (2013) A behavioural analysis of fleet driver safety, Driver Metrics blog post, 28 May 2013. Available at: www.drivermetrics.com/blog/behavioural-analysis-fleet-driver-safety/ [Accessed: May 2025].

Driver and Vehicle Licensing Agency (2025) Renew or change a lorry or bus licence. Available at: https://www.gov.uk/renew-lorry-bus-coach-licence [Accessed: May 2025].

Driver and Vehicle Licensing Agency (2024) Assessing fitness to drive. Available at https://assets.publishing.service.gov.uk/media/66c8b0d0e39a8536eac052f4/assessing-fitness-to-drive-august-2024.pdf [Accessed: June 2025].

Driver and Vehicle Standards Agency (2023) *The Official DVSA Guide to Driving: The Essential Skills*. London: The Stationery Office.

Hatakka M, Keskinen E, Gregersen N et al (2002) From control of the vehicle to personal self-control: Broadening the perspectives to driver education. *Traffic Psychology and Behaviour*, 5, 201–216.

HMSO (2025) *The Highway Code*. Available at: www.gov.uk/browse/driving/highway-code [Accessed: June 2025].

Police Foundation (2020) *Roadcraft: The Police Driver's Handbook*. London: The Stationery Office.

R v Cooksley and Others (2003) EWCA Crim 996.

Sharp G, Seagar H and George C (1997) *Human Aspects of Police Driving*. Glasgow: Road Safety Scotland.

UK Government (2025) Driving licences. Available at: https://www.gov.uk/browse/driving/driving-licences [Accessed: June 2025].

Further reading

Driver behaviour
A more detailed discussion on the topic of attitudes and driver behaviour can be found in blog posts by Dr Lisa Dorn of Cranfield University on www.drivermetrics.com

Lighting
Details of all legislation on lighting are available on the legislation.gov.uk website, which is managed by The National Archives on behalf of the government.

Legislation

The following legislation can be viewed in full at www.legislation.gov.uk:

Control of Pollution Act 1974
    Section 62

Corporate Manslaughter and Corporate Homicide Act 2007

Deregulation Act 2015

Health and Safety (Safety Signs and Signals) Regulations 1996

Health and Safety at Work etc. Act 1974

Motorways Traffic (England and Wales) Regulations 1982

Provision and Use of Work Equipment Regulations 1998

Road Safety Act 2006

Road Traffic Act 1988
    Sections 35 and 36

Road Traffic Exemptions (Special Forces) (Variation and Amendment) Regulations 2011

Road Traffic Regulation Act 1984
    Sections 5 and 87

Road Vehicles (Construction and Use) Regulations 1986
    Regulation 99
    Regulation 107
    Regulation 101

Road Vehicles (Construction and Use) (Amendment No. 2) Regulations 2005

Road Vehicles (Construction and Use) (Amendment No. 4) Regulations 2009

Road Vehicles Lighting (Amendment) Regulations 2005

Road Vehicles Lighting and Goods Vehicles (Plating and Testing) (Amendment) Regulations 2009

Road Vehicles Lighting Regulations 1989
    Regulation 24

Serious Organised Crime and Police Act 2005 (Consequential and Supplementary Amendments to Secondary Legislation) Order 2006

Traffic Signs and General Directions Regulations 2002
    Regulations 10 and 26
    Regulation 15(2)
    Regulation 26(5)(b)
    Regulation 27(3)(c)
    Regulations 33, 34, 35, 36(1)(a), 38(a/b)
    Regulation 36(1)(b) (red light)
    Regulations 47, 48, 49

Zebra, Pelican and Puffin Crossing Regulations and General Directions 1997

Index

www.ingramcontent.com/pod-product-compliance
Lightning Source LLC
Chambersburg PA
CBHW041145230326

41599CB00039BA/7180